Self-Assessment Color Review

Small Animal Dermatology

Volume 2: Advanced Cases

Karen A Moriello
DVM, DACVD
Department of Medical Sciences
School of Veterinary Medicine
University of Wisconsin–Madison, Wisconsin, USA

Alison Diesel
DVM, DACVD
Department of Small Animal Clinical Sciences
College of Veterinary Medicine and Biomedical Sciences
Texas A&M University, Texas, USA

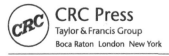
CRC Press
Taylor & Francis Group
Boca Raton London New York

CRC Press is an imprint of the
Taylor & Francis Group, an **informa** business

CRC Press
Taylor & Francis Group
6000 Broken Sound Parkway NW, Suite 300
Boca Raton, FL 33487-2742

© 2014 by Taylor & Francis Group, LLC
CRC Press is an imprint of Taylor & Francis Group, an Informa business

No claim to original U.S. Government works

Printed on acid-free paper
Version Date: 20130801

International Standard Book Number-13: 978-1-84076-197-9 (Paperback)

Visit the Taylor & Francis Web site at
http://www.taylorandfrancis.com

and the CRC Press Web site at
http://www.crcpress.com

Preface

The first edition of this book covered a general review of basic small animal dermatology. In this book, we have used the case-based and question format to present a review of advanced small animal dermatology. Also different from the first text is an expanded bibliography of references.

Karen A. Moriello
Alison Diesel

Acknowledgements

We would like to thank our colleagues for contributing cases in the following specialties.

Dermatology
Adam P Patterson DVM DACVD**
William Oldenhoff DVM*
Darcie Kunder VMD*

Internal medicine
JD Foster VMD*

Surgery
Jason A Bleedorn DVM DACVS*

Neurology/neurosurgery
Heidi Barnes Heller DVM DACVIM
(Neurology)*

Radiation therapy
Michael A Deveau DVM, MS,
DACVR (Radiation Oncology)**

Pathology
Aline Rodrigues Hoffmann DVM, MS,
PhD, DACVP***

* Department of Medical Sciences
School of Veterinary Medicine, University of Wisconsin–Madison, Wisconsin, USA

** Department of Small Animal Clinical Sciences
College of Veterinary Medicine and Biomedical Sciences, Texas A&M University, Texas, USA

*** Department of Veterinary Pathobiology
College of Veterinary Medicine and Biomedical Sciences, Texas A&M University, Texas, USA

Abbreviations

ACTH	adrenocorticotropic hormone	NSAID	non-steroidal anti-inflammatory drug
AD	atopic dermatitis		
ANA	antinuclear antibody	PAS	periodic acid–Schiff
ASIT	allergen-specific immunotherapy	PCD	plasma cell pododermatitis
		PCR	polymerase chain reaction
CBC	complete blood count	PF	pemphigus foliaceus
CDA	color dilution alopecia	PNU	protein nitrogen unit
CLE	cutaneous lupus erythematosus	PSOM	primary secretory otitis media
		RAST	radioallergosorbent test
CNS	central nervous system	RNA	ribonucleic acid
CPV	canine papillomavirus	SCC	squamous cell carcinoma
CsA	cyclosporine A	SIG	*Staphylococcus intermedius* group
CSF	cerebrospinal fluid		
CT	computed tomography	SLE	systemic lupus erythematosus
DIM	Dermatophyte Identification Medium	T_4	thyroxine
		TEN	toxic epidermal necrolysis
DLE	discoid lupus erythematosus	TEWL	transepidermal water loss
DLH	domestic longhair (cat)	Th	T helper (cell)
DMSO	dimethyl sulfoxide	TNF	tumor necrosis factor
DNA	deoxyribonucleic acid	TSH	thyroid-stimulating hormone
DSH	domestic shorthair (cat)	VCAM	vascular cell adhesion molecule
DTM	dermatophyte test medium		
EDS	Ehlers–Danlos syndrome	VCLE	vesicular cutaneous lupus erythematosus
ELISA	enzyme-linked immunosorbent assay		
EM	erythema multiforme		
FeLV	feline leukemia virus		
FIV	feline immunodeficiency virus		
FNA	fine needle aspiration		
GABA	gamma-aminobutyric acid		
Gy	gray (radiation measurement)		
HA	hyaluronan		
IDT	intradermal skin test/testing		
Ig	immunoglobulin		
IL	interleukin		
IVIG	intravenous immunoglobulin		
kDa	kiloDalton (molecular weight measurement)		
MCT	mast cell tumor		
MIC	minimum inhibitory concentration		
MRI	magnetic resonance imaging		

Broad classification of cases

Allergic cases
1, 11, 13, 15, 17, 27, 38, 44, 59, 61, 62, 67, 74, 81, 106, 116, 134, 174, 184, 187, 188, 198, 242

Alopecic cases
4, 26, 29, 76, 94, 109, 121, 182

Autoimmune cases
19, 28, 40, 45, 52, 60, 83, 138, 142, 149, 151, 171, 185, 196, 199, 205, 210, 215

Bacterial cases
2, 10, 16, 34, 36, 37, 48, 50, 53, 66, 93, 98, 129, 146, 153, 158, 204, 217, 219, 233, 239

Congenital cases
107, 135, 209, 221, 227, 230

Diagnostic cases
14, 24, 25, 30, 68, 70, 77, 100, 104, 115, 127, 156, 189, 228, 231, 243, 244

Ear cases
9, 56, 97, 108, 132, 148, 150, 167, 203, 234, 238

Endocrine cases
39, 41, 79, 110, 112, 155, 157, 191, 245

Fungal cases
5, 33, 54, 120, 133, 145, 160, 162, 175, 176, 180, 210, 218

Keratinization cases
20, 46, 124, 143, 186, 197, 212, 235, 237

Metabolic cases
21, 57, 82, 90, 168

Miscellaneous cases
31, 55, 78, 84, 87, 105, 137, 147, 152, 161, 163, 165, 169, 177, 181, 183, 200, 207, 213, 214, 224, 226, 229, 240, 241

Neoplasia cases
7, 51, 92, 111, 118, 119, 122, 126, 128, 130, 178, 190, 201, 236, 246

Nutrition cases
42, 223

Parasite cases
12, 18, 22, 64, 71, 72, 73, 80, 89, 96, 101, 113, 136, 140, 141, 144, 159, 173, 179, 194, 195, 202, 211, 220, 222

Pigmentation cases
3, 23, 85, 88, 139, 166

Structure and function cases
58, 95, 114, 170, 172, 193

Therapy cases
6, 8, 32, 43, 49, 63, 75, 86, 91, 99, 103, 117, 123, 125, 131, 154, 164, 206, 208, 216, 225

Viral cases
35, 47, 69, 102, 141, 192

To my family – Mark, Ethan, and Doug
Thanks TEAM!

KAM

To Mike – for allowing me to be 'boring' and work too many late nights and evenings. This could not have been completed without the support and understanding of my wonderful family
– thanks Mom, Dad, and Erica for bearing with me through the holiday!

AD

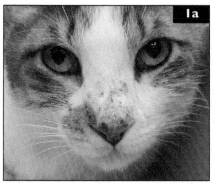
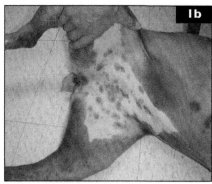

1 The owners of a dog and cat presented them in the morning for the complaint of acute onset of skin lesions overnight. The cat had lesions limited to the nose (**1a**) and the dog had lesions limited to the ventrum (**1b**). Close examination of the cat's nose revealed swelling and erythema of the haired area of the nose, multifocal areas of hair loss, and hemorrhagic crusts with small areas of focal erosion at the junction of the nasal planum and haired skin. Examination of the dog revealed a ventral distribution of lesions most noticeable in the thinly haired areas of the inguinal region. Skin lesions consisted of multifocal crusted papules surrounded by circular erythematous macules. The skin lesions were notably pruritic in the dog. When asked about the previous evening's activities, the owners reported that the dog and cat had spent the evening in their garden and yard, as usual.

i. Focusing just on the presentation of the skin lesions, what are possible differential diagnoses for the nasal lesions in the cat and the ventral skin lesions in the dog?

ii. Considering the clinical presentation of these patients, what is the most likely cause of the skin lesions? How can this be definitively diagnosed?

iii. What treatment do you recommend?

2 Bacterial cultures of the skin are necessary for the appropriate treatment of many skin infections.

i. What is the standard bacterium inoculum for testing antimicrobial susceptibility?

ii. Describe three techniques for determining the MIC of antibiotics. What is the 'breakpoint MIC'?

1 i. Cat: pemphigus foliaceus, dermatophytosis, demodicosis, atopy, food allergy, insect bite hypersensitivity. Dog: bacterial pyoderma, insect bite hypersensitivity, chigger bites, flea bites, purpura, vasculitis, erythema multiforme, drug reaction.
ii. Insect bite hypersensitivity, most likely mosquito, gnat, or *Culicoides* spp. These are most common in the evening. Definitive diagnosis requires keeping both pets out of the garden in the evening hours and observing resolution of the skin lesions followed by challenge exposure. This could be difficult as outdoor conditions vary. Wind, temperature, and humidity are factors affecting the presence or absence of insects.
iii. The lesions will resolve without treatment if repeated exposure is prevented. Topical therapy is difficult in cats and the lesions are not serious enough to warrant systemic glucocorticoid therapy unless they progress. The dog is pruritic; skin cytology is recommended to ensure bacterial overgrowth is not a complicating factor. Treatment is guided by cytologic findings, which in this case revealed no microbial overgrowth. The dog was treated with a topical glucocorticoid spray containing triamcinolone. Flea control products with permethrins designed to repel mosquitoes can be used in dogs to prevent recurrence. Permethrins are toxic to cats.

2 i. The standard inoculum is 10^5 colony forming units/ml of the bacterium.
ii. (1) Broth microdilution technique. Drug is added to medium in a 96-well microtiter tray and serially diluted to the desired drug concentration to be tested. The microorganism is then added and the tray incubated for 18–24 hours. The lowest concentration preventing visible growth is the MIC. (2) Agar dilution test (Kirby–Bauer, disk diffusion). Agar plates incorporating antimicrobial drugs at pre-determined drug concentrations directly into the medium are inoculated with a known concentration of the microbe directly onto the plate. Plates are incubated and again the lowest drug concentration inhibiting growth is the MIC. (3) E-test. The microorganism is inoculated over the entire surface of an agar plate and an E-strip containing gradients of drug concentrations is added to the surface of the plate and incubated. After incubation, the point on the E-strip that intersects the line of bacterial inhibition is the MIC. The breakpoint MIC is the highest drug concentration that can be achieved safely with clinically acceptable drug doses and routes of administration. Organisms are considered 'sensitive' if the MIC is well below the breakpoint, 'intermediately susceptible' if the MIC approaches the breakpoint, and 'resistant' if the MIC surpasses the breakpoint.

3 A 5-year-old female spayed husky dog presents for the lesions shown (3). The lesions are confined to the non-haired skin of the nasal planum and lips; no other skin lesions are present at examination. The owner reports that the dog is otherwise healthy, with the exception of its eyes 'looking a bit different' and it has been 'squinting' recently.

i. What are your differential diagnoses for this patient?

ii. What diagnostic testing is indicated?

iii. What is the most likely diagnosis for this patient?

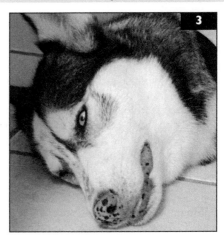

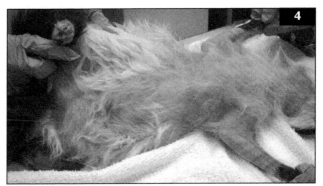

4 A 9-month-old male neutered cat is recovering from panleukopenia. The veterinary nursing staff report that the cat is shedding excessively (4). According to the staff, the cat is not pruritic. On examination, the cat is not 'shedding hairs', but rather the hairs are easily broken at the level of the follicular ostium.

i. What are the two major differential diagnoses?

ii. What diagnostic tests should you perform?

iii. Assuming the diagnostic testing is negative, what is your diagnosis and prognosis?

3 i. Lupus, uveodermatologic syndrome, idiopathic vitiligo, cutaneous epitheliotropic T-cell lymphoma, contact hypersensitivity, irritant reaction.

ii. Skin biopsy to differentiate among the differential diagnoses listed above. Given the concurrent involvement of an organ system other than the skin, skin biopsy is indicated sooner rather than later. A thorough ophthalmologic examination is needed to look for evidence of uveitis.

iii. Uveodermatologic syndrome. This is an immune-mediated disease that presents similarly to Vogt–Koyanagi–Harada syndrome in people. In dogs, the disease produces vitiligo and alopecia of the skin and mucosa along with granulomatous panuveitis. Histopathologic examination of skin biopsy specimens shows acanthosis of the epidermis, often with parakeratosis. Melanin in the basal layer is decreased or absent. Dermal inflammation is present as a perivascular to dense lichenoid infiltrate with the latter occasionally obscuring the dermal–epidermal junction. Ophthalmic changes can be severe and, if diagnosis is delayed, enucleation is often needed. Treatment includes immunosuppression (corticosteroids, cyclosporine, topical tacrolimus, azathioprine) and management of the uveitis. The condition has been reported in various breeds of dogs; however, Akita dogs appear to be most commonly affected. A recent study identified an increased frequency of a certain DLA class II allele (DQA1*00201) in American Akita dogs, which may be involved in the pathogenesis of uveodermatologic syndrome.

4 i. Dermatophytosis and anagen effluvium.

ii. Skin scraping and fecal flotation examination are needed to rule out feline demodicosis. *Demodex gatoi* is usually pruritic; the cat could be pruritic, but it was simply not observed. *D. cati* is often found in cats with systemic illnesses. Given that the hair breakage started suddenly and presumably the dermatologic examination was normal at the time of admission, dermatophytosis is unlikely, but a Wood's lamp examination and fungal culture are indicated.

iii. Anagen effluvium, which is very common in cats that have been severely ill or under other stressful situations (change of environment, surrender to animal shelter, poor plane of nutrition). In cats with severe upper respiratory infections, particularly kittens, the effluvium can start within a week of the event. Anagen effluvium will occur in young animals that have a large number of actively growing hairs; when the animal experiences a sudden illness, this will interrupt normal hair growth, making them fragile and easily broken. Hairs break when traction is placed on them, giving the impression that hairs are being shed. In telogen effluvium, anagen hairs rapidly progress to the telogen state as a bodily defense mechanism to conserve metabolic resources. Hairs are all synchronized in telogen and when new hair growth starts, hairs are shed in large numbers or patches.

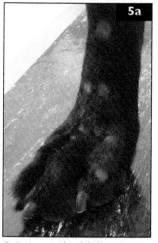

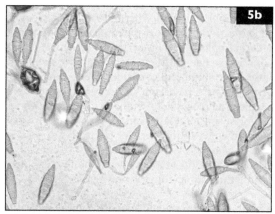

5 A 6-month-old dog is presented for multifocal areas of hair loss on the legs (5a), face, ears, and trunk. The lesions shown here are characteristic of others present over the dog's body. The dog lives outside in a dog pen; alopecia developed shortly after it started to dig holes in the ground. The dog is not reported to be pruritic.
i. What are the differential diagnoses?
ii. Initial diagnostic tests do not reveal a diagnosis and the owner declines treatment pending further results. A cytologic preparation from a pending diagnostic test is shown (5b). What is the diagnosis, how is this treated, and how do you explain the source of the infection?

6 Essential fatty acid (EFA) supplementation has long been a recommendation for the management of various inflammatory disorders in dogs and cats.
i. What is the difference between omega-3 and omega-6 fatty acids?
ii. What organs may be affected by the anti-inflammatory effects of omega-3 fatty acid supplementation?
iii. How have EFAs been utilized in the management of dermatologic conditions in dogs and cats?

5 i. Demodicosis, dermatophytosis, and bacterial pyoderma with or without secondary yeast overgrowth.

ii. *Microsporum gypseum* dermatophytosis. *M. gypseum* is a geophilic dermatophyte and infections often are inflammatory; the more inflammatory the reaction to a dermatophyte the faster the infection will self-cure. Ideal treatment includes both a systemic antifungal (itraconazole or terbinafine) and a topical antifungal rinse (lime sulfur, enilconazole). Dermatophytosis will self-cure, but the purpose of treatment is to hasten recovery and minimize contagion to other animals and people. The most likely source of infection is the dirt in the dog pen. Dogs that dig and/or spend large amounts of time outdoors exposed to soil are the ones most likely to contract this dermatophyte. There is no way of decontaminating the dog pen. In fact, little is known about how to control the organism in the environment. Decontamination attempts would only be reasonable if the dog continues to contract infection from the dog pen.

6 i. Omega-3 fatty acids (e.g. docosahexaenoic acid [DHA] and eicosapentaenoic acid [EPA]) are found in cold water fish (mackerel, cod), walnuts, and flaxseed. Omega-6 fatty acids are found in seeds and nuts and their extracted/refined oils. Gamma-linolenic acid (GLA) is an example of an omega-6 fatty acid; it is the precursor to dihomo-γ-linolenic acid (DGLA) as well as arachidonic acid. Fatty acids are a component of the phospholipid bilayer that comprises cell membranes; dietary intake of the various fatty acids will alter the composition of the cell membrane. Both omega-3 and omega-6 fatty acids compete for metabolic enzymes; activation of cell membrane phospholipases initiates an inflammatory cascade. Omega-6 fatty acids typically form pro-inflammatory mediators such as series 4 leukotrienes (e.g. B4) and series 2 prostaglandins (e.g. E2). Omega-3 fatty acids tend to form less pro-inflammatory mediators; series 3 prostaglandins (e.g. E3) and series 5 leukotrienes (e.g. B5) are formed instead.

ii. Include the skin, kidneys, gastrointestinal tract, neural tissues, cardiovascular system, and bones.

iii. EFA administration has been evaluated in dogs and cats with various inflammatory skin diseases including AD, cutaneous adverse reactions to food, and various feline cutaneous reaction patterns (miliary dermatitis, eosinophilic skin lesions). Various dosing regimens have been recommended, ranging from 35–90 mg/kg/day of combined DHA and EPA. Supplementation as part of or sole therapy for symmetrical lupoid onychodystrophy has also been reported.

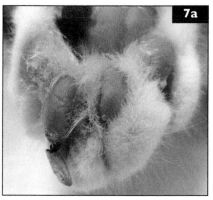
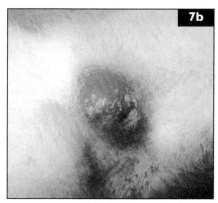

7 An 18-month-old female spayed Siamese cat was presented for evaluation of multiple abnormal claw growths involving all four feet. Multiple digits on each paw were affected as well as the metacarpal pads of both paws (**7a, b**).
i. What is this condition?
ii. What are the clinical features of this disease?
iii. Describe the etiology of the disease.
iv. What is the treatment of choice?

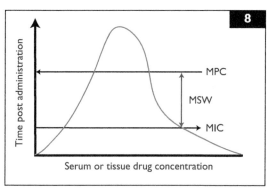

8 Define mutant prevention concentration (MPC) (**8**) and mutant selection window (MSW) and how these hypotheses relate to selection for resistant strains of bacteria. What weaknesses of minimum inhibitory concentration (MIC) values does the MPC hypothesis seek to correct?

7 i. Cutaneous horns.

ii. Cutaneous horn is a general term that describes a well circumscribed, conical or cylindrical mass of keratin. Lesions may be single or multiple and are firm on palpation. Trauma to the masses may result in localized hemorrhage. Lesions may vary from several millimeters to >2 cm in height. Lesions have been described in association with and in the absence of FeLV. Lesions are typically located in the center of digital, central, or metacarpal pads in cases of viral-associated cutaneous horns. In the non-viral form, masses may only form on digital pads just below the claw.

iii. Examination of the epithelium underlying the cutaneous horn is necessary to determine the etiology of the condition. Lesions may arise from viral papillomas, actinic keratosis, bowenoid in situ carcinoma, or invasive SCC. Virus isolation may be necessary to confirm or refute the presence of FeLV.

iv. Surgical removal. This may be accomplished via cryotherapy, laser removal, or classical surgical techniques. Owners must be alerted to the possibility of lesion recurrence. Based on the underlying cause of cutaneous horn development, prognosis is considered to be variable.

8 MPC can be defined as the MIC (minimal concentration of antibiotic that inhibits the growth of 10^5 colony-forming units) of the most resistant bacterial organism. For drugs such as fluoroquinolones, MPC can be defined as the antibiotic concentration that would require a microorganism to possess two simultaneous mutations at two different metabolic steps to grow in the presence of the antibiotic. Mutant subpopulations are typically present at low frequencies (e.g. 10^{-6} to 10^{-8}). In some infections, there may be several-fold more bacteria than the numbers used in standard MIC testing. As a consequence, it becomes likely that first-step mutants are present, thus selecting for resistant bacteria. These first-step mutants carry a single mutation conferring partial resistance to the antibiotic. The MPC hypothesis states that with higher concentrations of antibiotics, one can inhibit both susceptible and first-step resistant bacterial cells. MSW is the drug concentration range between the MIC and the MPC and can be thought of as the range that selects for first-step resistant organisms. One study found two distinct regions of growth inhibition when studying fluoroquinolone resistance patterns in higher density (>10^9) concentrations of bacteria. The first region of inhibition was approximated to the MIC. The second region, which completely blocked all growth, was termed the MPC. Between the MIC and the concentration of complete inhibition, viable bacteria could be isolated. These bacteria were found to have mutations that conferred resistance to the antibiotic being tested. Weaknesses of MPC include lack of standardization, lack of data, and the fact that MPC calculations are labor intensive. MPC is helpful only for bacteria that acquire resistance via mutations and not gene transfer.

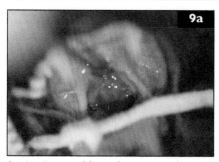

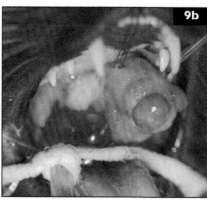

9 A 5-year-old male neutered DSH cat presented for a 3-month history of respiratory stertor. Physical examination

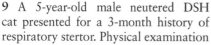

was unremarkable other than the previously mentioned stertorous breathing noted at rest. Otic examination was within normal limits. Sedated oral examination revealed the presence of a large, pink, soft tissue mass located dorsal to the soft palate (9a). Retraction of the soft palate with a snook hook allowed exteriorization of the mass using a stay suture (9b).

i. What is this mass?
ii. What additional diagnostics and treatment are recommended for this patient?
iii. What complications are associated with treatment? What is the prognosis?

10 A 4-year-old female spayed Labrador retriever dog is presented for moderate pruritus. The owner describes an increase in licking and scratching, particularly along the ventral abdomen and flanks. The owner seems to remember a similar occurrence the previous year around the same time. On physical examination, you notice these lesions on the ventral abdomen (10). No other lesions are noted on the dog.

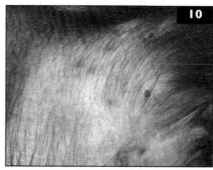

i. Describe the lesions seen on this patient.
ii. This is a common presentation of skin disease in dogs. What are three possible causes of the lesions seen?
iii. Of the possible etiologies, which is most common in the dog?
iv. What organism is isolated most commonly?

9 i. A feline nasopharyngeal polyp, the most common nasopharyngeal disease of younger cats and the most common non-neoplastic mass of the feline ear. Although the etiology is unknown, it is hypothesized that the polyps are congenital defects arising from remnants of branchial arches or are a response to irritation from chronic viral infections. Histopathologically, these masses contain a core of loose fibrovascular tissue covered by a stratified squamous to ciliated columnar epithelium with variable inflammatory infiltrates. Viral PCR for feline herpesvirus 1 or feline calicivirus has failed to substantiate the tissue persistence of these viruses in inflammatory polyps.

ii. Diagnostic imaging can be performed under heavy sedation or general anesthesia to further localize the polyp and determine if involvement of the bulla exists. Conventional skull radiographs of the bulla include right and left lateral oblique and open mouth rostrocaudal views, but these often lack sensitivity and are compromised by superimposition of the bones of the skull. Cross-sectional imaging using CT and MRI are complementary imaging studies of the middle ear and auditory canal and their contents; they are superior diagnostics for diseases of the ear. CT provides excellent images of bony structures and is indicated where osseous changes are of greatest diagnostic importance. MRI is superior in imaging soft tissue components including fluid and soft tissue density within the middle ear. Removal of the polyp is recommended by either simple traction/avulsion or ventral bulla osteotomy (VBO).

iii. Traction/avulsion of the polyp is considered if adequate grasp of the polypoid stalk is possible; however, the recurrence rate approaches 33%. Polyps without evidence of bulla involvement may be arising from the Eustachian tube, not the middle ear, allowing more complete removal of affected tissue via traction/avulsion. When bulla involvement is present, complete removal of affected tissue cannot be achieved without VBO. Surgical excision through VBO is recommended for definitive treatment and allows for complete removal of polyps and the epithelial lining of the bulla. Complications include Horner's syndrome, respiratory compromise, hemorrhage, seroma/hematoma formation, and recurrence. Features of Horner's syndrome include miosis, ptosis, enophthalmos, and elevation of the third eyelid; this occurs in up to 80% of cats postoperatively, although is often transient. Deafness is also reported in cats with nasopharyngeal polyps, although VBO does not appear to contribute to or provide resolution of hearing impairment as measured by air-conducted brainstem auditory evoked response.

10 i. Papules, pustules, and epidermal collarettes are noted along the ventral abdomen. Small erythematous macules may also be seen.

ii. These lesions are compatible with folliculitis. Common causes include bacterial pyoderma (superficial), demodicosis, and dermatophytosis.

iii. Bacterial pyoderma. Dermatophytosis, on the other hand, is the most common cause of folliculitis in the cat.

iv. *Staphylococcus pseudintermedius.*

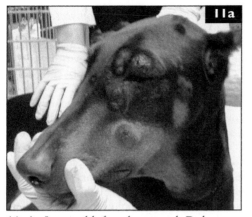
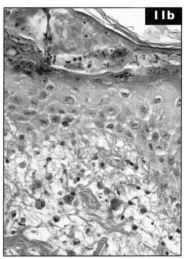

11 A 5-year-old female spayed Doberman pinscher dog presented on emergency because of an acute nodular eruption over

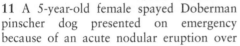

her head, face, and neck that had been persistent over 2 days (11a). Prior to lesion development, the dog had been running in the woods without owner supervision. On physical examination, there were numerous cutaneous, fairly firm nodular lesions, some as large as 3 cm in diameter, located multifocally over the head, face, and neck. Facial swelling was also noted, particularly along the muzzle and periocular region. A serous exudate was present from the center of several nodules; others were covered by a dried, adherent crust.

i. List the differential diagnoses.

ii. A biopsy from one of the nodular lesions is shown (11b, 40x). Histopathologic findings showed several intracorneal and subcorneal vesicles and vesicopustules containing low numbers of inflammatory cells, including neutrophils and eosinophils. Spongiosis and exocytosis of neutrophils and eosinophils were noted throughout the epithelium. There was intense edema in the subjacent dermis and marked superficial hemorrhage. A perivascular to interstitial infiltration with neutrophils and eosinophils was present. The histopathologic diagnosis was 'severe neutrophilic and eosinophilic vesiculopustular dermatitis; severe diffuse eosinophilic and neutrophilic dermatitis with marked vascular reactivity'. Based on this description, how is the differential list changed?

iii. What is the pathogenesis of urticaria and angioedema?

iv. What are common triggers of urticaria and angioedema in the dog?

12 How much blood can an actively feeding female cat flea (*Ctenocephalides felis*) consume?

11 i. Infections (bacterial: atypical *Mycobacteria, Nocardia, Actinomyces*, botryomycosis, L-form bacteria; fungal: blastomycosis, histoplasmosis, cryptococcosis, coccidioidomycosis), inflammatory processes (urticaria and angioedema, eosinophilic furunculosis, eosinophilic cellulitis, cutaneous histiocytosis, sterile pyogranuloma/granuloma syndrome), neoplasia (mast cell tumor, cutaneous lymphoma).

ii. Urticarial allergic reaction, contact hypersensitivity reaction, eosinophilic cellulitis. Culture is necessary to rule out bacterial infection (negative). Urticarial allergic eruption, insect bite reaction, and contact hypersensitivity reaction were considered most likely.

iii. Mast cell (or basophil) degranulation causes release of histamine, leukotrienes, and prostaglandins. These chemokines cause increased vascular permeability and smooth muscle contraction, causing an immediate (type I) hypersensitivity reaction. Release of IL-4 from mast cells and/or basophils causes Th2 cell differentiation and activation, leading to elevations in eotaxin and VCAM, thereby increasing tissue eosinophils, basophils, and Th2 cells. This causes a later phase inflammatory response. Type III hypersensitivity reactions may also be involved in urticaria development along with non-immunologic triggers that may precipitate or intensify the presence of lesions.

iv. Various drugs and chemicals, vaccines, food or food additives, stinging or biting insects, plants, bacterins, physical forces (pressure, cold, heat, sunlight, exercise), physiologic stress, genetic abnormalities. Infusion of human serum albumin has been associated with both acute anaphylactoid reactions and delayed development of urticaria and angioedema in dogs.

12 An average of 13.6 microliters of blood per day or approximately 15.15 times their body weight. A heavy infestation of fleas could easily cause anemia in a puppy or kitten. For example, a 0.5 kg kitten has approximately 30 ml of blood. An infestation of 220 female fleas could potentially consume 10% (3.0 ml) of the kitten's blood per day.

13 A 2-year-old male castrated Persian cat presented for intense facial pruritus with exudation (**13**). The cat had been obtained from a rescue organization 1 year previously. Dermatologic abnormalities at the time had been mild, limited to occasional serous ocular and nasal exudation with staining and debris on the face. Pruritus at the time of adoption was mild; however, it had progressed continuously until the time of presentation. The owner reported

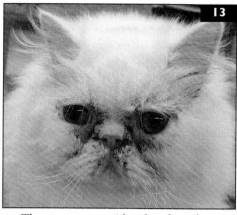

minimal response to antibiotic therapy. The cat was considered to be otherwise healthy, although it did have a history of intermittent sneezing and mucoid nasal discharge. On dermatologic examination, there was moderate conjunctivitis and periocular swelling with serous to slightly mucoid exudation adhered to the face, neck, perioral, and periocular regions. Moderate erythema was present along the medial aspects of the pinnae, periocular, and facial skin. Dark debris was present within both external ear canals and facial folds. The facial folds were noted to be more severely erythematous, moist, and abraded.

i. What is the list of differential diagnoses for this patient?

ii. What diagnostic tests do you recommend for this patient?

iii. A skin biopsy specimen was obtained from the affected skin on the muzzle. Biopsy results showed severe acanthosis with spongiosis of the epidermis, occasional to sparse individual keratinocyte degeneration (apoptosis), and a thick serocellular crust. There were numerous mast cells, moderate neutrophils, and a few eosinophils infiltrating the superficial dermis. Sebaceous hyperplasia was also noted. Given the clinical appearance, breed, and diagnostic findings, what is the most likely diagnosis for this patient?

iv. What is the underlying etiology of the condition?

v. What secondary complications are noted with the condition?

14 Specimens for bacterial culture and susceptibility or cytologic examination are easily collected from pustules. How do you collect specimens for culture and/or cytology from pyoderma lesions when pustules are not present?

13 i. Dermatophytosis, demodicosis, *Malassezia* dermatitis, bacterial folliculitis, cutaneous adverse reaction to food, environmental allergies, primary seborrhea, facial dermatitis of Persian and Himalayan cats. Given the history of sneezing and nasal discharge, upper respiratory infection (e.g. calicivirus, herpesvirus, *Mycoplasma*) should also be considered.

ii. Deep and superficial skin scrapings (negative); impression cytology (several cocci bacteria and yeast, occasional neutrophils, ceruminous debris); ear swab cytology (excessive ceruminous debris, no organisms); fungal culture for dermatophytes (negative); possible treatment trial for mites (*Notoedres cati* and *Demodex gatoi*), possible hypoallergenic diet trial based on other test results. Additional diagnostics could include intradermal or serum allergy testing, skin biopsy, *Mycoplasma* PCR, viral isolation, and transtracheal wash.

iii. Facial dermatitis of Persian and Himalayan cats.

iv. This condition is suspected to have a hereditary or genetic basis. Facial dermatitis is uncommon to rare in both Persian and Himalayan cats. It presents initially in older kittens or young adult cats and tends to progress in severity over time. Adherent debris, presumed to be sebaceous gland material, is a striking feature of the disease; a defect in cornification is suspected. Lesions are typically confined to the muzzle, periorbital region, and chin. In the initial stages of disease, pruritus may be absent to mild. As the disease becomes chronic, intense pruritus is often reported.

v. Secondary infections with bacteria and/or *Malassezia* yeast are common and may increase the severity of clinical signs. Submandibular lymphadenopathy has been reported in affected cats.

14 Look for areas of crusts and gently lift the crust with a sterile instrument to collect bacterial culture specimens and/or cytologic specimens (**14**). Crusted lesions with erythema often have areas of moist exudation beneath crusts at the periphery. If no such lesions can be found, bacterial cultures can be obtained from 'dry' lesions. If this is necessary, moisten the tip of the sterile culturette within the transport medium and then vigorously rub it over the site. Rotate the swab to ensure that any organisms are inoculated onto the surface of the swab. Ideally, the microbiologist will rotate the swab as it is being inoculated onto the surface of the culture plate; routinely doing this will minimize false 'no growth' reports due to poor laboratory techniques. Cytology

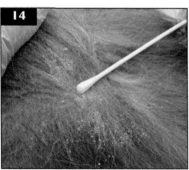

specimens can be collected from these sites using either clear acetate tape or impression smears. The latter is often difficult to do if the skin cannot be manipulated.

15 How is facial dermatitis of Persian and Himalayan cats (see case 13) treated?

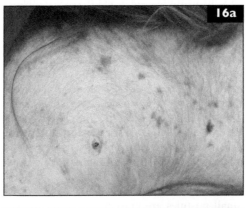

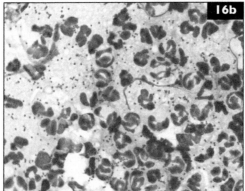

16 A 1-year-old female spayed golden retriever dog presented without any previous history of dermatologic abnormalities. The owners had taken the dog swimming over the weekend and noted these lesions on the dog's ventrum early Monday morning (16a). The dog had been mildly pruritic over the weekend, with pruritus concentrated along the ventrum where the lesions were present.

i. How would you describe the lesions seen?

ii. What are the differential diagnoses for the lesions?

iii. Cytology from a ruptured papule is shown (16b). What is the diagnosis?

iv. What is the recommendation for treatment?

15 Various treatment options have been evaluated, but no specific therapy has been determined. Therapy is aimed at treating secondary infections (antibiotics and/or antifungal medications) and minimizing the frequency of recurrence. Various topical products/shampoos have been evaluated to minimize and remove adherent debris (4% chlorhexidine, 2.5% benzoyl peroxide, 2% miconazole/2% chlorhexidine, other antiseborrheics); however, in most cats that permitted the washing, debris accumulated again within 1–3 days of therapy. Corticosteroid administration (prednisolone; periodic injections of repositol methylprednisolone acetate) partially controlled pruritus in some cats. Anecdotally, cyclosporine may be beneficial in some cats. A recent case reported successful management of facial dermatitis in a Persian cat with topical tacrolimus applied twice daily. Further evaluation of this option in more cats is necessary to determine the overall efficacy for management. In this case, cyclosporine (modified) showed fair treatment efficacy. The cat initially required concurrent administration of prednisolone (1 mg/kg q24h) to manage the intense pruritus; this was discontinued after 2 weeks. A protective Elizabethan collar was applied by the owner to help minimize self-trauma.

16 i. Papules and small pustules are present along the intertriginous skin of the ventral abdomen.
ii. These lesions are consistent with folliculitis. Common causes include bacterial pyoderma (superficial), dermatophytosis, and demodicosis.
iii. Superficial bacterial pyoderma.
iv. Since this is the dog's first episode of skin disease and the lesions are so diffuse, treatment should focus on resolving the current infection. An empiric systemic antibiotic may be prescribed; cephalexin would be a reasonable consideration since this is a large-breed dog. If the owners are unable to medicate the dog orally, cefovecin could be an alternative choice. This injection would need to be repeated in 7–14 days. Bathing with an antiseptic shampoo (e.g. ethyl lactate, chlorhexidine) would be a good adjunct therapy to help remove any adherent debris, aid in antimicrobial control of the organisms, and get the owners involved in disease monitoring. Bathing would be recommended 2–3 times weekly.

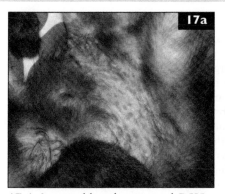
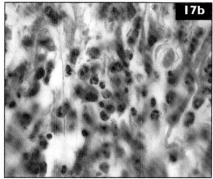

17 A 2-year-old male castrated DSH cat presented with a history of the lesions shown (17a). The cat was noted to be excessively pruritic with self-induced alopecia due to over grooming present along the ventral abdomen and medial aspects of both hindlimbs. The lesions responded well to corticosteroid administration; however, the owner was concerned about continued administration of these drugs and the young age of the cat. The cat lived strictly indoors and received year-round monthly topical flea prevention. Administration of several courses of antimicrobial treatments (antibiotics, antifungals) at adequate doses and duration did not lead to complete lesion resolution. Multiple strict hypoallergenic diet trials (commercial hydrolyzed and novel protein diets) had been attempted, but did not result in any decrease in pruritus. Biopsy of the lesions had been performed by the referring veterinarian (17b).
i. What are the lesions shown?
ii. This lesion has been associated with underlying allergic disease in cats. What other reaction patterns have been associated with feline AD?
iii. What are the options for long-term management of this cat?

18 An indoor/outdoor cat has a compound fracture of the femur of unknown duration. The wound at the site of the fracture is putrid and exudative, and the hair coat matted. Close examination of the wound reveals extensive myiasis.
i. What is the etiology and pathogenesis of myiasis?
ii. How will you manage the wound?

17 i. Eosinophilic plaques.
ii. Self-induced alopecia, head and neck pruritus, miliary dermatitis, eosinophilic lesions (eosinophilic plaques, eosinophilic granulomas, and indolent ulcers).
iii. Medical management or pursuing allergy testing with the goal of starting ASIT. Medical therapeutic options in cats are different to those in dogs. Topical bathing and topical antipruritics are common recommendations for pruritic dogs, but many cats do not tolerate bathing or topical products. Fatty acids and antihistamines may be helpful as adjunct therapy. Oral liquid modified cyclosporine for cats is well tolerated; adverse effects are similar to those seen in dogs, with gastrointestinal upset reported most commonly. The other option is to pursue allergy testing and ASIT administration. Serum allergy testing is often recommended initially in cats with a presumed diagnosis of AD since IDT may not be widely available and tests in cats can be more difficult to interpret. Cats often have less distinct wheals, which are softer and less erythematous than those found in dogs or people. If serum *in-vitro* test results are negative and AD is still suspected, IDT should be pursued. Injection of fluorescein dye may improve visualization of reactions; however, the usefulness of this is inconsistent. ASIT appears to be beneficial in approximately 50–75% of cats with a clinical diagnosis of AD.

18 i. Myiasis is infestation of tissues by fly larvae of the order Diptera. It is a disease of neglect or inattention. Adult flies lay eggs in open wounds, on moist skin, and on soiled hair coats (e.g. feces and/or urine), particularly in debilitated and recumbent animals. Larvae (maggots) hatch and secrete proteolytic enzymes that liquefy tissue and can create full-thickness damage within hours.
ii. Stabilize the patient, treat for shock and infection, identify the underlying neglect cause, kill/remove larvae, clip and clean the wound. Nitenpyram is a water-soluble neonicotinoid that is rapidly absorbed and rapidly excreted by the host; it has low toxicity for mammals. Within 20 minutes of administration, it reaches serum concentrations sufficient to act against insects. The most common use is for flea control. Recently, dogs with spontaneously occurring screw worm myiasis were treated with nitenpyram and within 1–2 hours of administration, 86% of larvae were spontaneously expelled. Dogs received a second dose 6 hours later and larval expulsion continued for 18 hours. Administration of nitenpyram as soon as myiasis is detected allows for larval kill to start before mechanical removal can be done humanely and safely. This can be administered rectally (off-label use) in animals too debilitated to swallow. Concurrent systemic treatments that can be used once the patient is stable include ivermectin, selamectin, and imidacloprid and moxidectin.

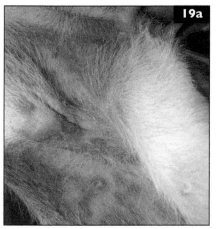

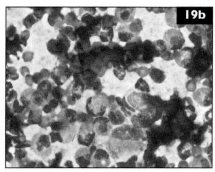

19 This 6-year-old male castrated Great Pyrenees dog was presented for skin lesions of approximately 2 weeks' duration (**19a**). The owner reported marked pruritus at the lesion site and in the axillary area; scratching had led to self-induced excoriations with serous exudate matting the hair. On physical examination, the dog appeared otherwise healthy except for the dermatologic abnormalities, but was notably pruritic during the examination when lesions were manipulated. The ventrum (mostly abdomen and inguinal region) had diffuse follicular and non-follicularly oriented pustules with erythematous margins. Large epidermal collarettes with erythematous margins and erosions were present. Some of the lesions appeared targetoid. The head was unaffected. The mucous membranes and non-haired skin were unaffected.

i. What are your differential diagnoses for this patient?
ii. What would you recommend regarding diagnostic work-up?
iii. Cytology from an intact pustule is shown (**19b**). CBC showed moderate to severe peripheral eosinophilia. Serum biochemistries did not reveal any significant abnormalities. Based on these findings, what is your diagnosis?

20 An extreme example of a common dermatologic lesion is shown (**20**).
i. What is this lesion called?
ii. What is the proposed pathogenesis?
iii. How can it be managed?

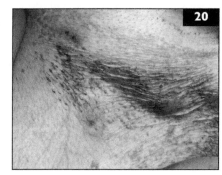

19 i. Superficial spreading pyoderma, superficial bacterial folliculitis, pustular drug eruption, dermatophytosis, demodicosis, sterile eosinophilic pustulosis, subcorneal pustular dermatosis, PF, CLE, neoplasia (cutaneous lymphoma, mast cell tumor).

ii. Deep skin scrapings to look for *Demodex* mites, cytology from the most active lesions, fungal culture, and bacterial culture and susceptibility. Since autoimmune diseases are on the list of differentials, infectious causes must be ruled out prior to treating the patient with immunsuppressive drugs. Biopsy may be necessary depending on the results of initial diagnostics (e.g. if parasitic, bacterial, or fungal organisms are not identified). CBC and serum biochemistries should be considered if warranted by the screening diagnostic tests. In general, CBC and serum biochemistries are not high-yield tests for strictly dermatologic diseases.

iii. Cytology revealed large numbers of eosinophils, which is not a common finding in bacterial pyoderma. A peripheral eosinophilia was noted. These preliminary findings are consistent with a diagnosis of sterile eosinophilic pustulosis. They should be confirmed with histopathologic analysis (biopsy will show superficial and subcorneal pustules containing large numbers of eosinophils; deeper hair follicles may also be affected) and negative bacterial and fungal cultures. This is a rare immune-mediated skin disease in the dog.

20 i. A comedone.

ii. Comedones are common in dogs and cats, but little is known about their pathogenesis. In people, comedones result from abnormalities in proliferation and differentiation of ductal keratinocytes. Comedones result from retention of hyperproliferating ductal keratinocytes; this has been confirmed by ^{3}H-thymidine labeling and an increase in Ki-67 labeling of ductal keratinocytes in comedone lesions. In addition, there is an increase in the presence of keratins 5 and 16 (keratin markers of hyperproliferation). Ductal hyperproliferation can result from abnormal sebaceous lipid composition, androgens, local cytokine production, and bacteria.

iii. Close inspection of the lesions reveals that many comedones are open; topical treatment could encourage evacuation of contents. Warm packing of the lesion for 5–10 minutes followed by gentle washing in clockwise and counter-clockwise directions will gradually evacuate lesions. Treatment of this area with topical retinoids or benzoyl peroxide will also help. Manually evacuating lesions via pressure (i.e. squeezing) should be strongly discouraged to prevent follicular rupture, development of deep pyoderma, and foreign body reaction.

21 A 6-year-old spayed female dog presented to the emergency service for vomiting, lethargy, and bloody diarrhea, as well as ecchymoses and petechiae on various skin surfaces. Approximately 2 weeks' prior, the dog was diagnosed with an open pyometra. At that time, an ovariohysterectomy and prophylactic gastropexy were performed in the same surgical procedure. The dog was discharged and cephalexin (30 mg/kg q12h), meloxicam (0.1 mg/kg q24h), and tramadol (3–4 mg/kg q8–12h) were prescribed. At the time of presentation to the emergency service, CBC showed decreased platelet count and mild left shift, and serum chemistries showed hypoalbuminemia (16 g/l [1.6 g/dl]; range 26–40 g/l [2.6–4 g/dl]). Clotting times were within reported normal ranges for the diagnostic laboratory.

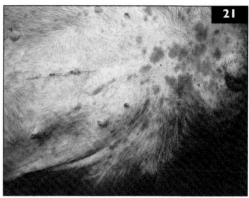

Skin lesions consisted of marked petechiae and ecchymoses on the ventral abdomen and inguinal region, which extended to the medial thighs (**21**). Lesions appeared targetoid and slightly raised in some locations. New pustular lesions were present around the mammae and ventral thorax. There was severe chemosis and conjunctival hemorrhage in both eyes and the muzzle was mildly edematous. Petechiation and small ulcers were present on the oral mucous membranes.

i. What are your differential diagnoses for this patient?

ii. Skin biopsy report showed 'patchy dermal hemorrhage with perivascular neutrophilic dermatitis affecting superficial and periadnexal vessels. The main change is edema, congestion, and areas of focal microhemorrhage. There is no fibrinoid necrosis to suggest vasculitis. In the worst affected areas there are large numbers of extravasated eosinophils and neutrophils in the perivascular dermis. Inflammation affecting the periadnexal vessels contains a large number of marginating leukocytes, chiefly neutrophils and eosinophils'. How do these biopsy findings relate to the patient's clinical presentation?

22 Approximately how many flea species have been identified? Summarize the general information known about the life cycle of the flea.

Answers: 21, 22

21 i. EM, drug reaction (antibiotics, NSAIDs), vasculitis/vasculopathy, warfarin poisoning.

ii. The extreme extravasation of leukocytes and edema noted in the biopsy samples is suggestive of 'leaky' blood vessels supplying the skin. The vascular integrity in this patient is compromised, leading to the petechiation and ecchymotic hemorrhages seen clinically. Decreased vascular integrity has been shown to be a consistent finding in human and animal patients with sepsis. The previous presentation for open pyometra likely contributed to systemic infection or inflammation, possibly related to endotoxemia. Similar skin lesions are seen in dogs that ingest garbage and develop endotoxemia secondarily. The endotoxemia reportedly causes increased chemotaxis of inflammatory cells, primarily eosinophils and neutrophils. The release of inflammatory cytokines from the eosinophilic granules (e.g. bradykinin, histamine, leukotrienes) induces increased vascular permeability ('leaky vessels') manifesting with extravasation of leukocytes. In this case, the cutaneous lesions are a reaction to a systemic process: development of sepsis and decreased vascular integrity.

22 Approximately 2,500 species. Fleas complete a full life cycle from egg to adult that includes several larval stages and a pupal stage. The time from egg to adult varies among species. Once on a host, adult fleas feed and mate. A blood meal is required to complete ovary development in female fleas. Eggs are laid in the hair or surroundings of the host. Depending on conditions, eggs hatch into larvae in 1–10 days; temperature and humidity are key factors. Larvae lack legs but have biting mouthparts. They pass through three instar stages of varying duration relative to temperature and humidity. They are free moving and feed on organic debris, including flea feces. Larvae are negatively phototactic (avoid light) and positively geotrophic (prefer downward movement); they hide in carpets, couches, organic material, or bedding. The last instar stage develops into a pupa, which develops inside a cocoon. The cocoon is sticky and rapidly becomes covered with external debris thereby protecting and camouflaging it. Pupae last for weeks, months, and even up to a year until a host arrives. Once the flea emerges, it seeks a host for a blood meal. Depending on the species, adult fleas live either in the host's habitat ('nest' fleas) or on the host ('body' fleas). Fleas are variably host specific; mammals that range usually do not have fleas of their own as opposed to animals that have dens or nests.

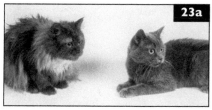

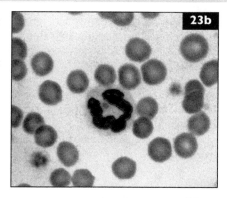

23 Two cats (23a) are presented for routine vaccinations. The owner reports that the cat with yellow eyes is clumsy, has 'twitchy eyes', and bleeds easily if injured. Physical examination of this particular cat reveals photophobia, nuclear cataracts, and prolonged nystagmus on intentional rotation.

i. What is the name of the coat color in these cats?

ii. A blood smear (23b) and a hair trichogram (23c) from the cat with yellow eyes are shown. What are the findings?

iii. What is the diagnosis?

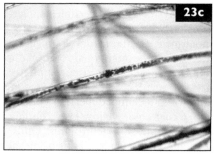

24 Infectious skin diseases can be diagnosed via cytologic techniques, histopathologic techniques, and microbial cultures. In addition, serologic tests can be used to detect antigens from an agent or an antibody response. In the last decade, molecular testing has become commercially available for the detection and diagnosis of many infectious agents. Molecular assays rely on the detection of RNA and DNA and consist of four nucleotides in varying sequences. Molecular testing takes advantage of the fact that many portions of DNA and RNA are conserved between organisms, whereas others are very specific to the organism on a family, genus, species, or even strain level. The sequence specificity is used to detect the organisms in clinical samples. Briefly describe the molecular detection of pathogens without DNA or RNA amplification.

23 i. Color dilution of the hair coat, often described as 'blue smoke' color.

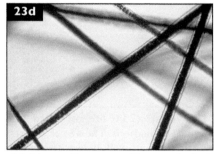

ii. Note the large intracytoplasmic vesicles (see **23b**) in the neutrophils. This cat was also neutropenic. The hair trichogram shows abnormally large melanin clumps (**23c**) within the hair shaft compared with normal hairs (**23d**).

iii. Chediak–Higashi syndrome. This is a primary immunodeficiency of cats, specifically Persian or Persian cat-crosses with blue and cream or blue smoke hair color and yellow eyes. The disease is genetic and is inherited in an autosomal recessive manner with complete penetrance. Cats are born with normal eyes, but by 28 days of age, irreversible changes in the tapetum are found; the structure is completely lost by 1 year of age. Cats can be described as 'clumsy' due to visual impairment as cataract development is common. Prolonged nystagmus is common after activity or intentional rotation during examination. Recurrent infections and abnormal bleeding can occur in affected cats. In a blood smear, neutrophils have large intracytoplasmic vesicles (lysosomes). Skin biopsy and hair trichogram show enlarged and clumped melanin granules. Diagnosis is made by clinical signs (blue smoke coat color, yellow eyes), finding of enlarged melanin granules in hair, and enlarged vesicles in neutrophils. Other hereditary causes of hypopigmentation in dogs and cats include albinism, piebaldsim, Waardenburg–Klein syndrome, and canine cyclic hematopoiesis of collie dogs.

24 The simplest molecular test for detecting infectious agents is a 'probe'. In this test, a complementary nucleic acid sequence is tagged with a fluorescent molecule to improve sensitivity. The probe is then added directly to the sample (fluid or tissue). Depending on the agent, multiple probes can be used on the same specimen for the detection of multiple infectious agents. This technique is rapid and easy to perform. Unfortunately, the sensitivity of this technique is not high compared with the sensitivity of other molecular tests. It can be improved with microbiologic culture, but this then requires knowledge of the culture requirements of the microbe and delays the testing results. This test is useful for slow growing organisms such as fungi or mycobacteria that are growing in the presence of other more rapidly growing organisms. It is also useful for rapid quantification of microbes in a sample. In-situ hybridization is a specialized type of probe applied to tissue. It allows for the detection of organisms in inflammatory lesions or in specific tissue in which the microbe might be part of a large number of organisms, many of which are normal flora.

25 What is real-time quantitative PCR (qPCR)?

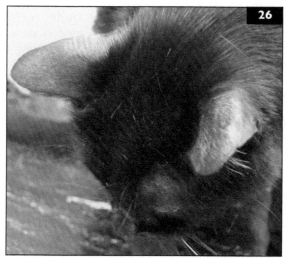

26 This 9-year-old cat (26) presented for the complaint of hair loss on the ears. The owners have pictures of the cat as a young adult and the ears are fully haired. Other than the noted alopecia on the ears, the dermatologic and medical examination was normal.

i. What is the most likely diagnosis?

ii. What are the causes of focal non-inflammatory alopecia in cats?

25 A technique that allows for both detection of the pathogen and the quantification of microbial load. The production of DNA during each amplification cycle is monitored so that the original quantity can be extrapolated by identification of the logarithmic amplification phase of each individual reaction. This technique uses fluorescent dyes or probes that produce a signal after formation of the product. During each cycle, a detector monitor records the amount of fluorescence in the sample. This assay has all the advantages of traditional PCR, but offers a more rapid result and can be used to quantitate the microbial DNA or RNA load. Problems with this assay are related to quality control; the use of dyes or fluorescent probes can lead to false-positive results. Quality control is dependent on the use of a published protocol and minimum laboratory standards. Problems occur when diagnostic laboratories use proprietary reactions not subject to independent validation and peer review.

26 i. Pattern baldness. Cats have two common presentations of non-inflammatory hair loss on the head: normal pre-auricular alopecia, which is most notable in darkly haired cats, and acquired pinnal alopecia. Skin biopsy shows small, atrophic hair follicles or total loss of hair. This is a heritable disease and is common in some breeds of cats (e.g. Siamese). It is important when presented with a case of pinnal alopecia to determine whether it is inflammatory or non-inflammatory. If inflammatory, issues such as coat color and symmetry become important in the diagnosis. Cats with light colored hair coats may have inflammatory pinnal hair loss due to solar exposure. Actinic changes and squamous cell carcinoma should be considered differential diagnoses. Actinic changes are most commonly bilateral, but they can be unilateral if the cat has 'sunburn' on one side of its face. The other major causes of inflammatory hair loss are dermatophytosis, PF, and insect bite hypersensitivity. Fungal culture, impression smears (bacteria, yeast, acantholytic keratinocytes [e.g. PF]), and skin biopsy may be needed. A cosmetic outcome can be problematic with skin biopsy. Take a representative sample as close to the base of the ear as possible. Full-thickness through and through samples are rarely needed.
ii. Post-traumatic alopecia, post-injection alopecia (e.g. glucocorticoids), post-spot-on flea control alopecia, pattern baldness, pre-auricular alopecia, traction alopecia, alopecia areata, anagen or telogen defluxion.

27 There are two routes for immunotherapy administration: injection and sublingual. What are the advantages and disadvantages for each route?

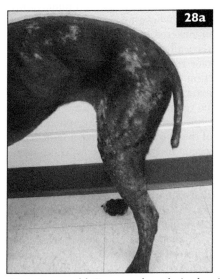 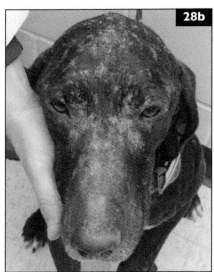

28 A 1-year-old German short-haired pointer dog was presented for the complaint of 'excessive dandruff' of several months' duration. The dog was also reported to be less active and reluctant to move at times; these clinical signs waxed and waned. The owner reported that one other littermate had similar clinical signs. Clinical examination revealed generalized exfoliative dermatitis over the entire body (28a, b). Follicular casts and thick adherent scaling were noted. No primary lesions were found. Skin scrapings were negative for *Demodex* mites, impression smears did not reveal bacteria or *Malassezia*, a fungal culture was negative, and there was no response to a trial of combined antimicrobial therapy for yeast and bacteria.

i. What are possible differential diagnoses?

ii. A skin biopsy was performed and the following findings were noted: orthokeratotic hyperkeratosis with moderate to diffuse interface dermatitis, mild to moderate apoptosis, and a lymphocytic interface mural folliculitis. A CBC revealed anemia and thrombocytopenia, ANA was negative, and direct immunofluorescence testing revealed IgG deposition at the epidermal basement membrane. What is the most likely diagnosis? What is the treatment and prognosis?

27 ASIT can be administered via subcutaneous injections or via sublingual immuno-therapy (SLIT). The latter has been used in people for many years and is considered safe and efficacious. Recently, SLIT has been evaluated in house dust allergic dogs and found to be safe and effective; it is currently a treatment option for ASIT in veterinary patients. The cost of allergen prescriptions can be comparable depending on dispensing practices. The major advantage of SLIT is that it eliminates the 'needle' and offers a therapy option for patients whose owners do not want to give injections. SLIT therapy needs to be administered twice daily every day. Care must be taken to position the pump vial vertically for proper allergen delivery. Side-effects are minimal; oral discomfort (face rubbing) and diarrhea have been reported. Allergen administration via injection is less time-consuming after the induction period. Local and major anaphylactic reactions have not been observed with SLIT in dogs; this may be a benefit or be yet undetermined since this therapy has only recently been introduced. Local allergic reaction post allergen injection is common and consists of pruritus at the site of the injection. Urticaria, angioedema, and generalized anaphylaxis are rare, but occur often enough to warrant client education.

28 i. The young age of onset and the fact that one other littermate was affected suggests a possible congenital or hereditary skin disease. The widespread distribution of lesions, history of waxing and waning, and clinical signs of systemic illness suggest the underlying etiology may be metabolic or immune mediated. Generalized exfoliative dermatitis in a dog <1 year of age in which other littermates may be affected is most compatible with ichthyosis or a primary disorder of keratinization; however, clinical signs of systemic illness are not associated with either disease. The young age of onset and the breed of dog make metabolic diseases such as zinc deficiency, vitamin A responsive disease, or superficial necrolytic dermatitis unlikely, as these scaling diseases are typically found in older dogs. Breed-related CLE is one possible explanation as this would account for other affected littermates and concurrent systemic signs of illness. Demodicosis is a considered differential diagnosis until ruled out via deep skin scrapings.
ii. Exfoliative CLE of German short-haired pointer dogs. Treatment is palliative and dogs show variable response to prednisolone, cyclosporine, hydroxychloroquine, and adalimumab. Topical treatment with keratolytic/keratoplastic shampoos and emollient therapy is helpful. Ultimately, the disease progresses and most dogs are euthanized by 4 years of age.

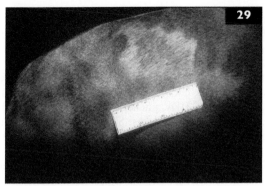

29 A young adult, female spayed boxer dog is presented for isolated hair loss along the left lateral flank (**29**). Alopecia began about 2 months previously and has progressively worsened. Pruritus or clinical signs associated with a systemic disease are not reported by the owner. Results of skin scrapings and skin cytology do not provide any definitive information.

i. List probable differential diagnoses based on the signalment, pattern of alopecia, and test results.
ii. How will you obtain a diagnosis?
iii. What is the most likely diagnosis for this focal hyperpigmented patch of non-pruritic alopecia on the flank?
iv. Is there an effective treatment for this condition?

30 Special stains are frequently used in histopathology to better identify a particular disease or disease process. They may be used to identify infectious organisms or highlight characteristics of various tissue types. The properties of each stain are variable; picking the correct stain for aiding in a diagnosis requires knowledge of the various stains available. What are the tissue-staining characteristics for the following special stains?

i. Periodic acid–Schiff.
ii. Brown–Brenn or Gram's.
iii. Gomori's methenamine silver.
iv. Verhoeff–van Gieson.
v. Masson trichrome.
vi. Alcian blue.
vii. Toluidine blue.
viii. Fite's.
ix. Sudan Black B.
x. Orcein–Giemsa.

29 i. Dermatophytosis, hypothyroidism, injection-site alopecia, canine recurrent flank alopecia (CRFA), alopecia areata, possible cutaneous reaction to topically administered steroids.

ii. Dermatophytosis can be excluded by fungal culture. Serum total thyroxine (TT_4) concentration along with the history and physical examination can assess thyroid function. Illness (sick euthyroid syndrome) and drug administration (e.g. sulfa antibiotics, steroids, NSAIDs, phenobarbital, clomipramine) can affect TT_4 interpretation, leading to a misdiagnosis. Skin biopsy from an area of maximal alopecia is needed to exclude other differentials.

iii. Given the signalment, distribution of alopecia, and lack of systemic signs, CRFA is most likely. CRFA (also known as seasonal or cyclic flank alopecia) is an uncommon form of recurring follicular dysplasia. Affected dog breeds include boxers, English bulldogs, schnauzers, and Airedale terriers. Well-circumscribed, usually hyperpigmented patches of 'geographical' or polycyclic-shaped alopecia develop focally or bilaterally along the flanks. This cyclic behavior may occur regularly or sporadically, or happen only once. Repeated episodes may eventually result in permanent alopecia. Skin biopsy shows dysplastic, atrophic, dilated, keratin-filled hair follicles with poorly formed secondary follicles extending into the surrounding dermis, and increased melanin deposition in adnexa.

iv. In some instances, oral melatonin (3–12 mg/dog q8–24h) will result in new hair growth within 2 months. Once new hair growth is observed, melatonin can be discontinued. If therapy is effective, it can be given pre-emptively several weeks before the next regularly recurring episode. Since this condition is considered a cosmetic disorder that may resolve spontaneously, generally no treatment is required.

30 i. Glycogen, neutral mucopolysaccharides, fungi, basement membrane = red.
ii. Gram-positive bacteria = blue; gram-negative bacteria = red.
iii. Fungi, melanin = black.
iv. Mature collagen = red; immature collagen, keratin, muscle, nerves = yellow; elastin, nuclei = black.
v. Mature collagen = blue/green; immature collagen, keratin, muscle, nerves = red.
vi. Acid mucopolysaccharides (e.g. mucin) = blue.
vii. Acid mucopolysaccharides, mast cell granules = purple.
viii. Acid-fast bacteria = red.
ix. Lipids = green-black.
x. Elastic tissue = black-brown; hemosiderin = green-black; melanin = gold-yellow; smooth muscle = light blue; collagen = pink; mast cell granules = metachromatic/purple; amyloid, cytoplasm of many cells = light or dark blue (dependent on cell type); nuclei = dark blue.

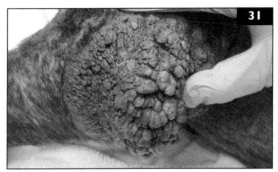

31 This lesion (31) is present bilaterally on the olecranon of a mastiff. On palpation, the lesion is fluctuant. What is it, and how is it treated?

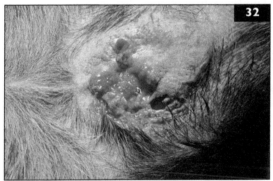

32 A 6-year-old German shepherd dog-cross presented for straining to defecate and licking the perianal region. On physical examination, numerous fistulous draining tracts were found in the perianal region (32). The dog was examined under sedation and it was determined that the fistulae did not communicate with the rectum and did not involve the anal glands. Oral anti-inflammatory drugs were prescribed, but discontinued due to severe gastrointestinal upset.
i. What class of drug is tacrolimus?
ii. What is the mechanism of action for tacrolimus?
iii. What formulation is used most commonly in veterinary medicine?

31 A hygroma complicated by marked hyperkeratosis. A hygroma is a false bursa that develops over bony prominences and pressure points, especially in large breeds of dogs. The most common cause is repeated trauma from lying on hard surfaces. This creates inflammation, which eventually results in development of a dense-walled, fluid-filled cavity containing yellow to red fluid. Clinically it presents as a soft, fluctuant, fluid-filled, painless swelling but in long-standing cases, ulceration, infection, abscesses, granulomas, and fistulae may occur. In addition to the hygroma, the skin becomes hyperkeratotic and proliferative. In general, hygromas are better prevented rather than managed; however, not all dogs will be cooperative and sleep on soft bedding. If the lesions are small, they can be managed via aseptic needle aspiration, followed by corrective housing. Soft bedding or padding over pressure points is imperative to prevent further trauma. Surgical drainage, flushing, and placement of Penrose drains are indicated for chronic hygromas. Areas with severe ulceration may require extensive drainage, extirpation, or skin grafting procedures. Use of intralesional corticosteroids is not recommended. In this case, the 'feathering' hyperkeratosis acted as a reservoir of microbial overgrowth, preventing any type of surgical intervention. The lesion was managed with daily bathing using an antibacterial–antifungal shampoo.

32 i. Calcineurin inhibitor.
ii. Tacrolimus (previously known as FK-506) binds to FK-506 binding protein in the cytoplasm of T cells. The complex inhibits calcineurin from dephosphorylating nuclear factor of activated T cells (NFAT), thus preventing it from being translocated into the nucleus. The inhibition prevents transcription of various inflammatory cytokines including IL-2, IL-3, IL-4, and TNF-α. Decreased inflammatory cytokine synthesis results in decreased activation and proliferation of helper and cytotoxic T cells.
iii. Although tacrolimus exists as an injectable and oral formulation, the latter of which is noted to be approximately 10 to 100 times more potent than cyclosporine, the topical formulation is used most commonly in veterinary medicine. Topical tacrolimus is available as a 0.03% and 0.1% ointment. Most clinicians prefer the 0.1% ointment unless the patient is not able to tolerate it due to discomfort. The topical ointment does not have systemic side-effects, making it useful for the treatment of localized disease. A common adverse effect reported by people is a mild burning or tingling sensation. A study evaluating the use of topical tacrolimus for treatment of perianal fistulae in dogs did not note post-application inflammation as determined by the dog's behavior (i.e. licking).

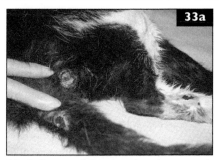
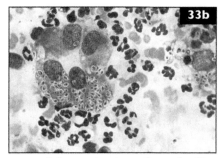

33 A 2-year-old indoor/outdoor cat is presented for evaluation of non-healing wounds on the face, legs, and trunk (**33a**). The lesions had initially been treated as cat bite abscesses with antibiotics at the correct dose and duration. Cytologic findings of an impression smear are shown (**33b**).
i. What is the diagnosis in this case?
ii. What diagnostic tests can be used in cats and dogs?

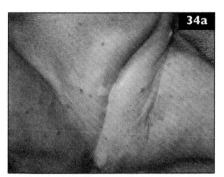
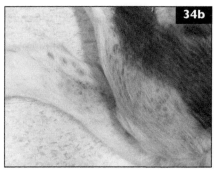

34 Two dogs are presented for superficial bacterial pyoderma (**34a, b**). One had an infection caused by a susceptible strain of *Staphylococcus pseudintermedius*, while the other had an infection caused by methicillin-resistant *Staphylococcus pseudintermedius*. Which one is which?

33 i. Sporotrichosis. *Sporotrix schenckii* is a dimorphic fungus that exists in mycelia form at 25–30°C and yeast form at body temperature (37°C). It has worldwide distribution but is most common in tropical and subtropical climates. Sporotrichosis is zoonotic; reports of transmission from cats to people have increased. In 2004, an epidemic was reported in Rio de Janeiro over a 6-year period in which 1,503 cats, 64 dogs, and 759 people had a diagnosis confirmed by isolation of the organism via culture. Infection in people was associated with cats with either clinical or non-clinical disease in 91% of cases. In 68% of human cases in this series, exposure was via bites or scratches.

ii. Fungal culture, cytology, histopathology, PCR, and immunofluorescence. For fungal culture, submit tissue wedges or exudate from deep inside the lesion. Cytologic diagnosis in cats can be made by examining tissue aspirates or impression smears. Seventy-nine percent sensitivity has been reported in a study comparing cytology and culture. In contrast, the sensitivity in dogs is much lower (32%) with these diagnostics; smaller numbers of organisms are present in the exudate of dogs. Histologic specimens should be obtained from new nodular lesions. The sensitivity of histologic examination when compared with culture is 62%. Two ELISA tests for feline sporotrichosis have been developed; when compared with culture from known cases they were reported to have a sensitivity and specificity of 90% and 96% (specific molecule test) and 96% and 98% (crude exoantigen), respectively.

34 Clinically, it is not possible to distinguish methicillin-susceptible from methicillin-resistant staphylococcal skin infections. The only way to determine this is with aerobic culture and susceptibility testing. It is important to remind the diagnostic laboratory (especially if it is not a veterinary specific diagnostic laboratory) to speciate the staphylococcal bacteria; both *Staphylococcus aureus* (primary pathogen in people) and *Staphylococcus pseudintermedius* (primary pathogen in dogs and cats) are coagulase-positive staphylococcal organisms. The implications for zoonosis are necessary information with regard to client education and patient handling. In general, *Staphylococcus pseudintermedius* does not readily colonize or cause infections in people; however, infections have been reported in people due to this organism, but it is not common. Colonization with this organism may be more common in people within the veterinary profession.

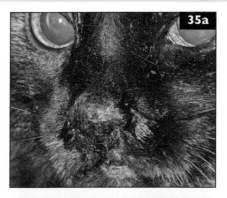

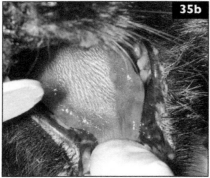

35 A 9-month-old stray cat was presented for examination because of the complaints of anorexia, fever, mild lethargy, and facial lesions (35a). Oral examination revealed these lesions (35b). What are the differential diagnoses?

36 Prior to infection developing, bacteria must adhere to and colonize the skin. If the environmental and source factors are right, then infection will subsequently occur. This process has been evaluated in species including dogs, cats, and people.
i. What is known about the degree of bacterial adherence to the skin of dogs, cats, and people?
ii. What is known about the mechanisms involved in the adherence and colonization of the skin by bacteria in dogs?

35 Feline upper respiratory disease (most likely), in particular feline herpesvirus (FHV) and feline calicivirus (FCV). Without any additional history, the differentials for the facial lesions alone include, but are not limited to, trauma, neoplasia, allergies, insect bite hypersensitivity, viral upper respiratory disease (herpes, calici) and immune-mediated diseases.

Skin lesions associated with FHV and FCV are increasingly being diagnosed because of immunohistochemistry (IHC) and PCR. Dermatologic lesions of acute FCV infection include oral vesicles and ulcers, lip ulcers, ulcers of the nasal philtrum, and, on rare occasions, ulcers on the body, although the latter are rare. Chronic FCV infection has been implicated as one of the causes of progressive plasmacytic–lymphocytic proliferative or ulcerative gingivitis and stomatitis. An uncommon but highly virulent form of FCV (FCV-associated virulent systemic disease [VSD]) can result in death within 1 week. These cats can show facial lesions and paw edema, pyrexia, ulceration, icterus, and hemorrhage from the nose and in the feces. Many of the cats with FCV-associated VSD have been vaccinated, suggesting the disease is caused by a strain not associated with vaccination. In FHV, skin ulcers and nasal dermatitis and stomatitis can occur and may have an eosinophilic infiltrate, making it a differential diagnosis for any ulcerative eosinophilic disease (i.e. 'eosinophilic granuloma complex'-like lesions). In one study, PCR testing was determined to be useful as an initial screening test, but due to false positives, IHC is needed to make a definitive diagnosis.

36 i. Feline corneocytes show reduced adherence of *Staphylococcus* species bacteria compared with either dogs or people. In a study evaluating *Staphylococcus* species from healthy individuals, feline keratinocytes were less likely to demonstrate bacterial adherence on an *in-vitro* model. *S. felis* was most adherent, followed by SIG, *S. aureus,* and *S. hominis.* Canine and human corneocytes demonstrated similar adherence profiles to each other. This finding may explain why cats tend to be 'more resistant' to development of bacterial pyoderma (or why their clinical manifestations of disease are different) as well as interspecies transfer of organisms compared with dogs and people, in which pyoderma is relatively common.
ii. In people, several bacterial surface proteins have been implicated in promoting adhesion to corneocytes. Clumping factor B is one such molecule. Cytokeratin 10 is a ligand implicated in bacterial binding. In dogs, *Staphylococcus* species bind to fibronectin, fibrinogen, and cytokeratin, suggesting that SIG bacteria, like *S. aureus,* possess an array of cell wall adhesins that allow them to recognize and bind various matrix proteins on the cells. Cell wall virulence factors possessed by *Staphylococcus* species bacteria also help mediate adhesion and colonization of skin. Two surface proteins (SpsD and SpsO) have been identified in *S. pseudintermedius,* which mediate binding and adherence to canine corneocytes. Others likely are present but await identification.

37 As discussed in case **36**, prior to infection developing, bacteria must adhere to and colonize the skin. How does underlying dermatologic disease factor into this process?

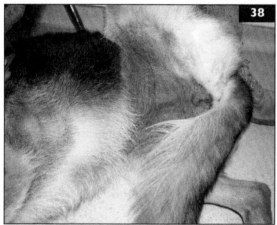

38 A 3-year-old German shepherd dog presented for recurrent pyoderma and chronic pruritus since 6 months of age (**38**). After a thorough work-up, the final diagnosis was recurrent bacterial and yeast pyoderma due to house dust and storage mite allergy. During discussion of immediate and long-term treatment options, the owner asks 'how do we get rid of the house dust mites?'.
i. What are the common house dust mites and storage mites?
ii. Where are these mites likely to be found in a home?
iii. What recommendations do you make to the client?

37 As with people, dogs with AD show a higher prevalence of *S. pseudintermedius* colonization (which may be reported by the diagnostics laboratory as 'SIG' since molecular testing is necessary to specifically identify *S. pseudintermedius*) of the skin compared with healthy counterparts. This degree of adhesion and colonization contributes to the higher frequency of skin infections in these canine patients. This is also true for people with AD. Similarly, it has been demonstrated that dogs with AD have an increased expression of antimicrobial peptides in the skin compared with non-atopic dogs; however, this expression is altered with regard to which antimicrobial peptides. For example, beta-defensin expression is different in dogs with AD compared with dogs lacking the disease. Although the amount of antimicrobial peptides is increased overall, the altered expression may also contribute to the development of secondary infections in atopic patients.

38 i. Dust mites: *Dermatophagoides farinae* and *D. pteronyssinus* are the most common species. Storage, mold, or grain mites: include *Acarus siro, Tryophagus putrescentia, Glycyphagus domesticus, Blomia tropicalis, Lepidoglyphus destructor.*
ii. House dust mites are found in pillows, mattresses, carpeting, upholstered furniture, and the dog's bed or bedding. Storage mites may be found outside food storage areas or in the environment. The prevalence of mites is dependent on environmental factors such as moisture and humidity. *D. farinae* is more tolerant of dryer climates than *D. pteronyssinus*. These mites feed on human skin scales, pollen, fungi, bacteria, and animal dander.
iii. House dust mites are found in all homes and are impossible to remove. An extensive review of house dust mite control measures for asthma found that intervention produced no significant difference in the number of patients that improved clinically, their asthma symptom scores, or medication use. Routine recommendations for control include: minimizing carpeting in the home; frequent washing of bedding; dusting; and thoroughly vacuuming several times a week. Electrostatic dusting cloths and filtered vacuums may be more effective at minimizing disruption of dust and hence dust mites. Pyriproxifen has been recommended as a method of controlling mites in the environment. Bathing to remove mites on the body and maintain the epidermal barrier function is practical. The allergic response is not just against live mites, but dead mite allergens as well; therefore, immunotherapy is recommended along with reasonable cleaning measures.

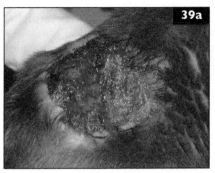
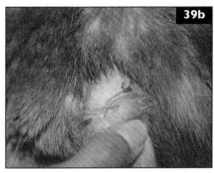

39 A 12-year-old female spayed DSH cat presented for a recent history of several cutaneous ulcers and erosions (39a). Minimal manipulation of the skin during examination revealed easily torn, fragile, thin skin (39b). The owner reported no other signs of systemic illness. The cat had a long history of non-seasonal moderate pruritus that had been well managed with corticosteroid administration.

i. What are the most common clinical signs associated with feline hyperadrenocorticism?

ii. How does iatrogenic hyperadrenocorticism differ in dogs and cats?

40 A 6-year-old male castrated Great Pyrenees dog presented for the clinical lesions shown (40). No other lesions are noted on dermatologic examination. Previous CBC and serum biochemistries performed by the dog's referring veterinarian did not reveal any abnormalities.

i. What is the most likely diagnosis in this patient?

ii. What are the options for treating this condition?

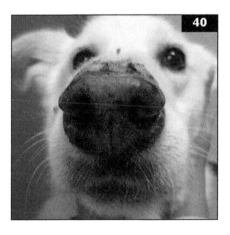

39 i. Physical findings may include: abdominal enlargement, muscle atrophy, thin skin, unkempt hair coat, hair loss (often bilaterally symmetrical), bruising, hepatomegaly, plantigrade stance, hyperpigmentation, and seborrhea. Skin fragility (skin that is easily torn with minimal handling or restraint) and curling of the ear pinnae are cutaneous side-effects seen exclusively in cats with hypercortisolemia; the latter is noted more frequently in iatrogenic hyperadrenocorticism compared with spontaneous disease. Most cats with hyperadrenocorticism have concurrent diabetes mellitus, typically insulin-resistant and difficult to regulate. Polyuria, polydipsia, polyphagia, lethargy, and increased frequency of upper respiratory and urinary tract infections may also be noted. Secondary bacterial pyoderma as well as generalized demodicosis is common.

ii. Compared with dogs, cats are noted to be less prone to side-effects of corticosteroid administration. Iatrogenic hyperadrenocorticism is much less common in cats, possibly due to the relatively low expression of corticosteroid receptors in cats compared with other species. Unlike dogs, cats may show signs of skin fragility and curled pinnae, as mentioned above. Alkaline phosphatase may be elevated; however, in cats this is a side-effect of poorly regulated concurrent diabetes mellitus as opposed to elevated cortisol. While dogs with hyperadrenocorticism show decreased urine specific gravity, cat urine typically remains concentrated (>1.030) despite concurrent polyuria and polydipsia.

40 i. DLE, pemphigus erythematosus, CLE, or neoplasia. A skin biopsy is needed to confirm the diagnosis.

ii. Numerous treatment options are available for DLE and pemphigus erythematosus in dogs depending on disease severity. Since the condition is restricted to a single body region, topical therapy may be considered to minimize systemic adverse effects. Potent topical steroids (e.g. betamethasone valerate, betamethasone dipropionate) may be used in severe cases in the initial stages to put the condition into remission. Caution must be used with this treatment option because of the high possibility for cutaneous atrophy. Alternatively, topical tacrolimus may be used to control the disease. Cutaneous atrophy is not a side-effect with tacrolimus as opposed to topical steroids. In more severe cases, systemic therapy may be indicated at least initially. Options would include immunosuppressive doses of corticosteroids (prednisone or prednisolone), cyclosporine, or combination therapy with tetracycline/doxycycline and niacinamide. A recent study in a dog has reported efficacy in treating a generalized variant of DLE with oral hydroxychloroquine. Additional research is warranted to assess this option for other lupus variants in more patients.

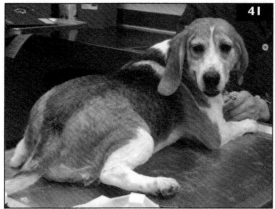

41 A 5-year-old male beagle dog was presented for the complaint of 'excessive shedding' of 4 months' duration (**41**). The dog had a lifelong history of primary seborrhea manifested by malodorous greasy skin with chronic recurrent infections/overgrowth of bacteria and yeast. Examination revealed easily epilated hairs, bilaterally symmetrical hair loss over the lumbosacral area, dry brittle hairs, superficial pyoderma, and malodorous seborrhea. A review of the medical records revealed that the dog had gained 6 kg since the last visit. Vital signs were within normal limits for a dog. Based on the history and clinical signs, hypothyroidism was suspected. A fasted serum chemistry panel revealed elevated cholesterol.

i. Hypercholesterolemia is a classic finding in dogs with hypothyroidism. In what other diseases is hypercholesterolemia a common abnormal finding on serum biochemistry panel?

ii. This dog has a lifelong history of recurrent bacterial and yeast pyoderma/overgrowth and seborrhea. What is the likelihood that these problems are due to the suspected hypothyroidism?

iii. What drugs might this dog have received that could interfere with thyroid function testing?

iv. What are the most common thyroid function tests, and what are their limitations?

Answer: 41

41 i. Cholestasis, hyperadrenocorticism, diabetes mellitus, nephrotic syndrome, post-prandial sampling, idiopathic hypercholesterolemia, familial hypercholesterolemia (schnauzers).

ii. If the dog truly has a lifelong problem with seborrhea that predisposes it to secondary microbial overgrowth, it is unlikely that this is due to hypothyroidism. Lifelong suggests the dog had the disease at a young age; dogs with hypothyroidism presenting at a young age would have congenital hypothyroidism and show signs of cretinism. The more likely scenario is that the dog has a primary disorder of keratinization and has developed breed-associated thyroiditis that exacerbated the pre-existing seborrhea and secondary microbial overgrowth.

iii. Glucocorticoids and sulfonamides. Glucocorticoids can decrease total T_4, free T_4, and TSH. They influence peripheral metabolism of thyroid hormones and inhibit TSH secretion. The effect is dependent on dose and preparation. Sulfonamides can decrease T_4 and free T_4, and increase TSH. They block iodination of thyroglobulin and can cause clinical hypothyroidism in a dose- and duration-dependent manner. Other drugs that can cause low T_4 include anticonvulsants, phenobarbital, NSAIDs, furosemide, phenylbutazone, radiographic contrast agents, general anesthesia, and previous levothyroxine therapy.

iv. Measurement of total T_4 in combination with clinical signs and serum chemistries can be used as a screening test. A normal total T_4 makes the diagnosis of hypothyroidism unlikely but not impossible. Sighthound dog breeds have normal total T_4 levels that are 50% lower than other breeds, therefore interpret with care. Free T_4 measured by equilibrium dialysis (FT_4ED) is less likely to be affected by most non-thyroidal illnesses and drugs and is not affected by autoantibodies. It has an approximate diagnostic accuracy of 90%; low test results are compatible with hypothyroidism, but also consider severe non-thyroidal illness, concurrent glucocorticoid or phenobarbital administration, or hyperadrenocorticism. Endogenous TSH is high in 60–80% of dogs with hypothyroidism and in 10–15% of dogs with non-thyroidal illnesses. The 'classic' hypothyroid dog has a low total T_4, low FT_4ED, and high TSH.

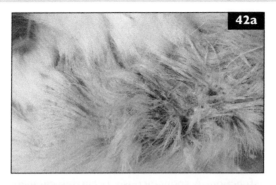

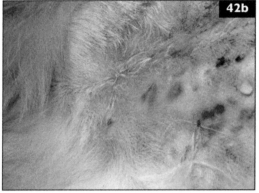

42 Nutrition, trace minerals, and vitamins play various roles in different aspects of skin health and disease. For each of the following vitamins, discuss their importance with regard to skin structure and function, and the disease states associated with vitamin abnormalities.
i. Vitamin A (**42a**)
ii. Vitamin B
iii. Vitamin C
iv. Vitamin D
v. Vitamin E (**42b**)
vi. Vitamin K

43 How was it discovered that a mutation in the *ABCB1* (*MDR1*) gene leads to increased toxicity to ivermectin?

42 i. Vitamin A is involved in cornification defects seen in cocker spaniel dogs. Compared with primary seborrhea, which presents at a young age, vitamin A-responsive dermatosis manifests in adults. Clinical signs include crusting, scaling, and alopecia. Follicular plugging, follicular casts, and frondlike keratinous debris are noted on the ventral and lateral thorax and abdomen.

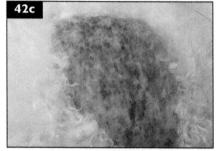

ii. In dogs and cats, vitamin B abnormalities are associated with neurologic and/or gastrointestinal dysfunction. A spontaneously occurring cutaneous manifestation of vitamin B deficiency has not yet been reported in small animals.

iii. Vitamin C is a cofactor in collagen synthesis. It is required by prolyl and lysyl hydroxylases for post-translational hydroxylation of procollagen. Vitamin C deficiency causes immature and insufficient collagen formation. Clinical signs include poor wound healing and dermal and capillary fragility.

iv. With solar exposure, the epidermis transforms provitamin D_3 into vitamin D_3 via previtamin D_3. It is translocated into the blood stream where it is hydroxylated in the liver (to 25-hydroxyvitamin D_3) and kidney (to 1,25-dihydroxyvitamin D_3). 1,25-dihydroxyvitamin D_3 is necessary in epidermal proliferation and differentiation.

v. Vitamin E is an antioxidant. Deficiency causes feline pansteatitis and is most commonly reported in cats fed exclusively a tuna diet or those supplemented with excess cod liver oil. Signs include widespread cellular damage and deposition of ceroid pigment. Nodules, typically without fistulation and drainage, are found in the subcutaneous and mesenteric abdominal fat.

vi. Vitamin K is a necessary cofactor for coagulation factors II, VII, IX, and X. Deficiency results in hemorrhage and spontaneous bleeding. Petechiae and ecchymotic hemorrhage may be easily visible on the skin and mucous membranes (**42c**).

43 In order to study the function of the *MDR1* gene, mice were developed that were homozygous for deletion mutations in the gene. The mice were viable and appeared phenotypically normal. However, when the colony became infested with mites, the mice were sprayed with a dilute ivermectin solution, which is normally considered to be a safe procedure. To the researchers' surprise, large numbers of mice were found dead shortly afterwards. Subsequent analysis revealed that all the dead mice were homozygous for the *MDR1* deletion (mdr1a -/-). Toxicity analysis demonstrated that the mdr1a-/- mice were 50–100-fold more susceptible to orally administered ivermectin than mdr1a+/+ or mdr1a+/- mice.

44 A 3-year-old female spayed golden retriever dog presented for moderate non-seasonal pruritus, mainly involving all four paws, face, ear pinnae, and ventrum, that had progressed in severity since the age of 8 months. The owners reported that clinical signs improved with the administration of anti-inflammatory doses of corticosteroids, but pruritus recurred once treatment was discontinued. Mild erythema of the affected body areas was the only abnormal finding on dermatologic examination. Multiple skin scrapings (deep and superficial) were negative for mites. Cytology did not show evidence of infection with either bacteria or yeast. Previous treatments for microbial overgrowth had not provided relief of pruritus according to the owner. There was no improvement following a miticidal treatment trial (for scabies) with ivermectin. No benefits were noted with regard to skin comfort following multiple strict hypoallergenic diet trials (hydrolyzed, multiple commercial novel protein diets). Both allergen-specific IgE serum tests and IDT were negative.

i. What is the definition of canine atopic-like dermatitis?
ii. What are the recommendations for medical management for this patient?

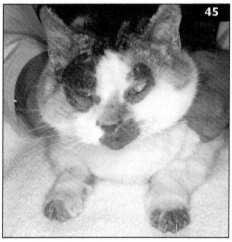

45 This cat was presented for the lesions shown (**45**). They had developed slowly over several months. What are possible differential diagnoses?

44 i. An inflammatory and pruritic skin disease with clinical features identical to those seen in canine AD in which an IgE response to environmental or other allergens cannot be documented.

ii. Very similar to those for dogs with documented IgE involvement; however, since the offending allergens are not able to be documented in these patients, ASIT is not part of the disease management. As with canine AD, avoidance of flare factors is a necessary part of long-term treatment. This includes an effective flea control program and antimicrobial therapy if signs of infection (bacteria or yeast) are present. Improving skin hygiene and coat care is also part of the management. Frequent bathing with a non-irritating or soothing shampoo, plus dietary fatty acid supplementation, is recommended. Topical glucocorticoids or tacrolimus may be beneficial for localized pruritus; however, systemic medication is often necessary for more widespread disease. Oral glucocorticoids, cyclosporine (modified), and subcutaneous interferon can help control clinical signs. When glucocorticoids are part of the management, steroid-sparing agents such as essential fatty acids or antihistamines may also be incorporated. As evidence for the involvement of epidermal barrier dysfunction in canine AD continues to accumulate, it is not unreasonable to suspect barrier dysfunction in canine atopic-like dermatitis as well. Improvements in barrier function may be more important for these patients if a 'leaky' epidermis takes precedence over immunologic disturbances with regard to disease pathogenesis.

45 The skin lesions shown are uncommon and not suggestive of a particular skin disease. Although unlikely, dermatophytosis needs to be considered, as it can mimic almost any known feline skin disease. Hair trichograms looking for demodicosis are indicated; however, if these mites are found, there is a strong possibility that demodicosis is secondary to an underlying disease. The marked symmetry of the lesions strongly suggests that the dermatologic lesions are a cutaneous marker of systemic illness or are immune mediated. Possible differential diagnoses include early epitheliotropic T-cell lymphoma, pseudopelade, sebaceous adentitis, follicular mucinosis, adverse drug reaction, SLE, and skin disease secondary to FIV. This is a case of follicular mucinosis, a rare, presumably immune-mediated skin disease that has been seen in association with cutaneous lymphoma in cats. Pseudopelade is a rare immune-mediated disease characterized by generally symmetrical alopecia that begins on the head and spreads to the legs, paws, and ventrum. Onychomadesis is a common finding. The alopecia tends to be non-inflammatory.

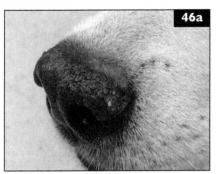
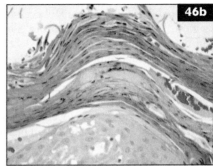

46 Note the nasal lesions in this crossbred Labrador retriever dog (46a).
i. What differential diagnoses would you consider if the owner reported that the onset of the lesions was rapid? What differential diagnoses would you consider if the lesions were reported to be slow in onset?
ii. A photomicrograph of a skin biopsy from the margin of the dog's nose is shown (46b). What key epidermal abnormality is shown?
iii. A complete dermatologic examination was performed and lesions were found to be limited to the planum nasale. The owner reports that the lesions began at approximately 6 months of age and have slowly progressed over the last several years. What is the most likely diagnosis?

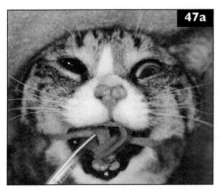
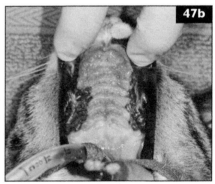

47 A farm cat was presented for a lesion on its nose (47a). The lesion was reported to have started slowly and is not painful. Examination under general anesthesia revealed more extensive lesions (47b). A skin biopsy was obtained and the lesion was identified as a 'feline sarcoid'. What is known about this disease?

46 i. Rapid onset: pemphigus foliaceus/erythematosus, lupus erythematosus, drug reaction, hepatocutaneous disorder. Slow onset and progression: zinc-responsive skin disease, nasal hyperkeratosis, ichthyosis in healthy younger dogs. In either situation it is important to examine the dog for lesions on other parts of the body, in particular the foot pads.

ii. Parakeratotic hyperkeratosis. Diffuse parakeratotic hyperkeratosis is most commonly seen in parasitic infestations, zinc-responsive skin diseases, lethal acrodermatitis, *Malassezia* dermatitis, hepatocutaneous syndrome (necrolytic migratory erythema, superficial necrolytic dermatitis), and breed-related nasal digital hyperkeratosis.

iii. Nasal parakeratosis of Labrador retriever dogs. This is a hereditary disease of Labrador retriever and Labrador retriever-cross dogs. Typically, lesions begin to develop between 6 months and 1 year of age and start as dry, rough, proliferative adherent keratin on the planum nasale. The disease is believed to have an autosomal recessive mode of inheritance. Histologically, parakeratotic hyperkeratosis is a striking feature. Nasal digital hyperkeratosis occurs in middle-aged to older dogs, whereas Labrador nasal parakeratosis occurs in young dogs. Zinc-responsive skin diseases usually are not limited to the nose. Inherited zinc-responsive skin disease (type I) occurs in northern breeds of dogs (e.g. Akitas, Malamutes, Huskies). If zinc-responsive skin disease caused the lesions in this dog, it would be most likely related to dietary deficiency (type II). Immune-mediated diseases would not progress this slowly and would damage the nasal planum and/or adjacent nares.

47 Feline sarcoids are rare skin tumors of cats. They can occur on the philtrum, nares, lip, digits, ears, and tail. They are more common in male cats from rural areas. They have been reported in domestic cats, bobcats, Florida panthers, Asian lions, snow leopards, and clouded leopards. They are usually solitary, slow growing, and may be locally infiltrative. Typical histologic findings include non-encapsulated, poorly demarcated dermal nodules that may invade the epidermis. The lesions need to be differentiated from spindle cell tumors such as fibroscarcomas, histiocytic sarcomas, and melanomas. The lesions are caused by a feline sarcoid-associated papillomavirus (FeSarPV). This virus has been detected in lesions in cats from both the USA and New Zealand. The virus is presumed to be of bovine origin and recently FeSarPV has been detected within bovine skin. This suggests that cattle may be the reservoir host of this virus and feline sarcoids are a 'dead end' infection by a bovine papillomavirus. Lesions often recur after surgical excision. Cryotherapy, radiation, or amputation has been used for permanent resolution of lesions.

48 A 13-year-old male castrated golden retriever dog presented for acute and rapidly progressive skin lesions involving the right forelimb. The owner had noted the dog limping on the limb 1 week prior to presentation; no traumatic injury had been observed. The dog was presented on emergency, was febrile (40°C [104°F]), tachycardic, and painful on palpation. The entire right forelimb was clipped and the full extent of the lesions was noted (**48a, b**). Multiple draining tracts were evident with purulent–hemorrhagic exudate oozing from the tracts and matting the surrounding hair. There were irregular patches of black tissue, which were extremely painful, surrounded by erythema and edema extending from the ventral neck to the carpus. Cytology of the exudate showed large numbers of bacterial organisms (cocci with occasional rods) with large numbers of neutrophils and occasional macrophages.

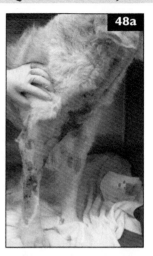

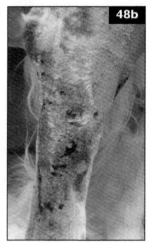

i. Because of the clinical appearance, aggressive surgical debridement was recommended along with culture and biopsy of the affected tissue. On surgical exploration, the subcutaneous tissue and deep fascia could easily be separated by gentle manipulation with one finger. What is the clinical suspicion given the lesion and surgical appearance?

ii. What organisms have been associated with this disease development in dogs?

49 Ketoconazole, itraconazole, fluconazole, and terbinafine are antifungal drugs commonly used in veterinary dermatology. What is the spectrum of activity of each drug with respect to fungal infections, and what are the common adverse effects in dogs and cats?

48 i. The discoloration associated with the lesions on the limb is tissue necrosis. This may have developed due to thrombus formation, chemical irritant (does not fit with the dog's history) or other reason for tissue devitalization (e.g. blunt trauma, infection). Systemic signs combined with the lesions lend concern for toxic shock syndrome or necrotizing fasciitis. Surgical findings are key; based on easily separated tissue, the dog was diagnosed with necrotizing fasciitis. Also known as 'flesh eating disease', this rare condition is caused by rapidly spreading bacterial infection leading to soft tissue damage. Most dogs have a history of even mild trauma, but this may not be required for disease development. Infection spreads, migrating through fascial planes, and involves deep tissues; ischemic necrosis from vasoconstriction and/or thrombosis leads to clinical lesions.

ii. The most commonly implicated bacterial organism in dogs is group G *Streptococcus* species (e.g. *Streptococcus canis*); this is the organism most commonly involved in canine toxic shock syndrome. Other reports have involved *Escherichia coli* and *Staphylococcus pseudintermedius*. Methicillin-resistant *Staphylococcus aureus* has been reported in association with necrotizing fasciitis in people due to virulence factors associated with this organism. There is suspicion that *S. pseudintermedius* may have similar virulence factors and should be considered a potential causative agent in this disease in dogs.

49
- Ketoconazole. *Candida, Malassezia, Blastomyces, Histoplamsa, Coccidioides, Cryptococcus*, less effective against *Sporothrix* and *Aspergillus*. Can be used for dermatophyte infections but itraconazole, fluconazole and terbinafine are preferred. Can cause anorexia, vomiting, diarrhea, abdominal pain, weight loss, hepatotoxicity. Do not use in cats as it is not well tolerated.
- Itraconazole. *Cryptococcus, Candida, Blastomyces, Histoplamsa, Coccidioides, Malassezia, Aspergillus, Sporothrix*, zygomycosis, chromomycosis, fungal keratitis, onychomycosis, dermatophytosis. It can cause vomiting, diarrhea, abdominal pain, inappetence, increased serum liver enzymes, fever, hypertension, skin rash, and ulceration.
- Fluconazole. *Cryptococcus, Candida, Blastomyces, Histoplamsa, Coccidioides, Malassezia*, variable efficacy against dermatophytes and *Aspergillus*. It can cause vomiting, diarrhea, cutaneous eruptions, and hepatotoxicity (elevated transaminases, cholestasis, hepatitis), although much less than with ketoconazole or itraconazole.
- Terbinafine. Dermatophytes, some activity against *Sporothrix*. Low efficacy against yeast. It can cause vomiting, diarrhea, abdominal pain, and rarely hepatotoxicity.

50 What is the overall prognosis for the dog in case 48?

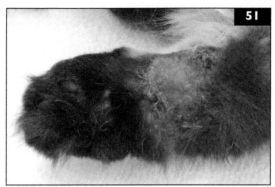

51 A 9-year-old DLH cat presented for a non-healing wound on the right hindlimb (51). The lesion had been present for several months without significant improvement noted by the owner. Systemic antibiotic administration had not provided any visible benefit to the patient. The cat resisted close examination of the lesion; however, it was noted to be a fairly well-circumscribed epidermal/ superficial dermal mass. The cat appeared somewhat painful on palpation. The owners also reported that the cat would groom excessively at the hindlimb. No other lesions were found on physical examination.

i. What are the differential diagnoses for the lesion seen on this cat?

ii. Biopsy of the mass revealed an unencapsulated mass involving primarily the superficial dermis, which was contiguous with the epidermis in several areas. Ulceration and erosion were present along the surface. The mass was composed of multiple, discrete aggregates of epithelial cells of variable size and shape. The cells were polygonal and occasionally had indistinct borders, with a high nuclear to cytoplasmic ratio. They were arranged in large lobules extending to the deep dermis; the lobules were composed of smaller variably sized nests and trabeculae separated by a small amount of fibrovascular stroma. Cell polarity was haphazard, particularly along the internal portion of the mass. The pathologist's note indicated that the appearance of the neoplastic cells resembled that of basal cells of the epidermis. Based on this description, what is the histopathologic diagnosis?

iii. How are these tumors in dogs and cats classified histopathologically?

iv. What is the typical behavior of these tumors in cats?

50 In general, the prognosis for necrotizing fasciitis in dogs is very poor. Fatality is common, particularly if the condition is not identified and addressed rapidly. Multiple surgeries, long-term antibiotic administration, and supportive care are indicated to give the patient the best chance. There is one report of successful management with a single surgical debridement; however, it is

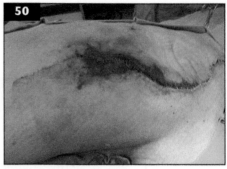

not the normal progression. In this case, the dog's right forelimb and surrounding tissue was amputated and thoroughly debrided. Approximately 1 week after the initial surgery, necrotic tissue was noted along the surgical site (50). A second aggressive, revisional surgery was performed to remove more of the devitalized tissue. The dog was provided with supportive care with appropriate antibiotic, fluid, and nutritional support for 3 weeks while he recovered. He was eventually discharged from the hospital, but was euthanized approximately 1 month following the procedure because of continued complications.

51 i. Non-healing wound with excessive granulation tissue (e.g. trauma, foreign body, infection); neoplasia; fungal granuloma; dermatophytic pseudomycetoma.
ii. Trichoblastoma (basal cell carcinoma).
iii. Into three different forms: solid, keratinizing, clear cell. Solid basal cell carcinoma is the most common variant noted in cats, whereas keratinizing carcinomas are most common in dogs. Clear cell basal cell carcinomas to date have only been reported in cats, but this variant is considered to be rare.
iv. Trichoblastomas are uncommon in cats and rare in dogs. Lesions are typically solitary, well-circumscribed plaques or nodules often with an ulcerated surface. Multicentric trichoblastoma appears to be more common in cats than dogs. Masses may have a blue or black pigmented appearance due to melanin pigment within the lesion. In cats, lesions are frequently located on the nose, face, and ears; truncal lesions are more common in dogs. In general, these tumors in cats have a very low rate of recurrence and metastasis. Analysis of nuclear morphology may be helpful in determining histologic subtype and predicting recurrence of tumor growth in cats with trichoblastoma; quantitative analysis of area, perimeter, and mean diameter of nuclei were found to be appropriate parameters in one study.

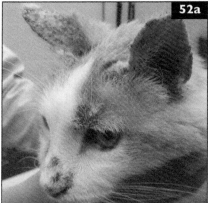

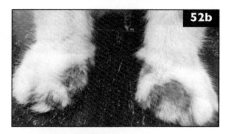

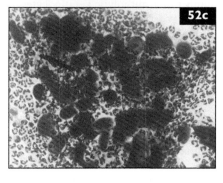

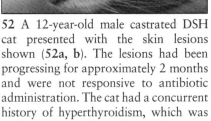

52 A 12-year-old male castrated DSH cat presented with the skin lesions shown (**52a, b**). The lesions had been progressing for approximately 2 months and were not responsive to antibiotic administration. The cat had a concurrent history of hyperthyroidism, which was well-managed with methimazole administration. No other signs of systemic illness were noted by the owner.

i. What are your differential diagnoses for this patient?
ii. Cytology from under the crusts/pustules is shown at 40x magnification (**52c**). What cytologic findings are noted?
iii. What is your most likely diagnosis for this patient?
iv. What treatment options are available for consideration?

53 A current topic in the veterinary literature is the increasing frequency of methicillin-resistant staphylococcal infections in animals. This trend is also seen in the human medical field. In dogs and cats, with regard to skin infections, *Staphylococcus pseudintermedius* is the most common isolate. This is different from people, in whom *Staphylococcus aureus* is most commonly isolated.

i. What does methicillin resistance mean?
ii. What implication does this have for public health?

52 i. Dermatophytosis, superficial bacterial pyoderma, PF, drug-associated PF or other drug reaction, subcorneal pustular dermatosis, eosinophilic pustulosis, cutaneous neoplasia (lymphoma, thymoma-associated exfoliative dermatitis), mosquito bite hypersensitivity.
ii. Large numbers of neutrophils (mostly intact and viable) with fewer eosinophils, lymphocytes, and macrophages; large numbers of acantholytic keratinocytes, often in groups or 'rafts'.
iii. PF and drug-associated PF are the most likely differentials due to the large number of acantholytic keratinocytes noted on cytology.
iv. The most commonly used and effective treatment options include glucocorticoid medication (prednisone, triamcinolone, dexamethasone) with or without adjunct non-steroidal medications. In some cats, a reasonably low dose of glucocorticoid alone may be sufficient to control the clinical signs of PF. In others, however, the addition of a non-steroidal medication (chlorambucil, cyclosporine) will allow for a more rapid and effective glucocorticoid dose reduction. In this case, treatment was initiated with prednisolone (4 mg/kg/daily for 10 days and tapered over several weeks). Methimazole was discontinued because of the potential for drug-associated PF. Radioactive iodine (I^{131}) was administered to control the cat's concurrent hyperthyroidism. Eventually, all treatment for PF was able to be discontinued without evidence of relapse.

53 i. Methicillin resistance in *Staphylococcus* species is due to an altered penicillin binding protein, PBP2a. This protein is unable to bind antibiotics with a beta lactam ring. This includes all penicillins, cephalosporins, and carbapenems. Methicillin is a semi-synthetic, penicillinase-resistant antibiotic. It is no longer produced; on susceptibility profiles, oxacillin (a more stable antibiotic) is used instead. Resistance to oxacillin is the same as methicillin resistance. Methicillin resistance is due to the presence of the *mecA* gene; *mecA* encodes for the altered penicillin binding protein. The *mecA* gene is carried on a staphylococcal chromosome cassette (SCCmec); this mobile genetic element becomes integrated into the *Staphylococcus* species genome. The cassette varies in size, but always contains the *mecA* gene. Also, it will frequently contain other genes responsible for antimicrobial resistance, thereby further limiting treatment options.
ii. The *mecA* gene responsible for methicillin resistance in *S. pseudintermedius* is the same gene that encodes for methicillin resistance in *S. aureus*. This has implication with regard to public health in that even though *S. pseudintermedius* does not readily colonize or infect people, the organism can potentially transfer the chromosomal cassette to *S. aureus* in a susceptible human carrier; resistance, therefore, can be transferred between species. The organism can persist in the environment for a fairly long period of time, lending concern for infection and/or colonization persistence or recurrence. This is true for both animals and people.

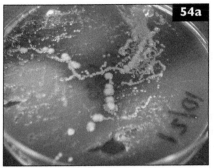
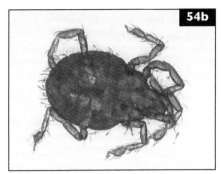

54 This is a DTM fungal culture plate inoculated 7 days ago (54a). Note the white glistening growth on the plate and how the microbial growth seems to have an irregular, if not serpiginous, growth pattern. An acetate tape preparation of the white growth was made and no evidence of bacteria, yeast, or fungi was found. Instead, this organism was found on the tape (54b). Close examination of other fungal culture plates in the same container revealed similar growth and tracks.

i. What is this organism?

ii. What is its source?

iii. How do you prevent other cultures from being contaminated?

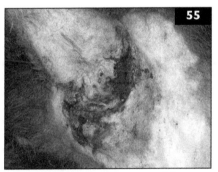

55 A 5-year-old German shepherd dog presents with presumed perianal fistulae (55). The owner reports the dog has difficulty defecating and is bleeding around the anus.

i. Name two other possible differential diagnoses.

ii. List other clinical signs dogs with perianal fistula may display.

iii. How is this treated?

54 i. A storage mite, which infests fungal culture medium. The two most common species are *Tyroglyphus* and *Tarsonemus*.
ii. Storage mites are usually brought into the laboratory on fresh materials and deposited onto the medium during inoculation of plates. The first indication of contamination may be moth-eaten fungal cultures or 'wandering trails of colonies' on the fungal culture medium. These mites not only eat the cultures, they will also carry fungal spores and bacteria from one culture to another.
iii. In clinical practice, prevention of infestation of in-house fungal cultures starts with sample acquisition. Inoculate samples quickly and discard any remaining specimens, store inoculated plates individually in self-sealing bags. If an infestation does occur, mites are very susceptible to environmental flea control products.

55 i. Anal gland abscess/rupture and perianal neoplasia. The former might be a confounding consequential factor with perianal fistulae.
ii. Hematochezia, dyschezia, obstipation, diarrhea, ribbon-like stool, increased frequency of defecation, perianal licking, self-mutilation, scooting, offensive odor, and/or weight loss.
iii. Perianal fistula is a relapsing and remitting disease; the disease is managed, but not necessarily cured. The first goal is to alleviate large bowel clinical signs (e.g. hematochezia, tenesmus, dyschezia). Reduction in the diameter, depth, extent, and recurrence of tracts/fistulae is the second goal. Medical management offers the best chance for resolution and consists of combined immunosuppressive/ immunomodulatory (e.g. glucocorticoids, calcineurin inhibitors, azathioprine), dietary (e.g. elimination diet, stool softeners), and hygiene (e.g. clipping, cleaning, antibiotics) therapy.

This disease is best managed medically; the most effective treatment has been cyclosporine. The 'modified' formulation of cyclosporine should be used as it is more bioavailable than earlier formulations. Although the use of an antimicrobial agent to reduce the cost of medical care with cyclosporine should be questioned, ketoconazole (8 mg/kg PO q24h) co-administered with CsA allows for an approximate 50% reduction in the dose. Ketoconazole is a P-450 enzyme inhibitor and reduces the metabolism of CsA. A tapering course of anti-inflammatory to immunosuppressive dosages of systemic glucocorticoids may be helpful. Once clinical signs have improved, especially pain, medical therapy can be transitioned from systemic to topical treatments. Tacrolimus (0.1%) ointment is applied twice daily and then slowly tapered to the most infrequent effective dose possible to maintain clinical resolution.

56 A 4-year-old female spayed Labrador retriever dog presented for unilateral otitis externa of approximately 7 days' duration. The dog was being treated for con-current immune-mediated thrombo-cytopenia of unknown underlying cause. The dog had a history of intermittent otitis externa, often with secondary *Malassezia* overgrowth, primarily in the warmer months when she spent a lot of time in the

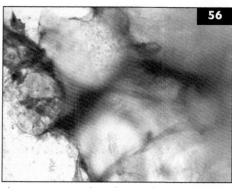

water. The owner had been cleaning the ear every other day with an acidifying cleaner; however, the ear appeared to be worsening. On otoscopic examination, the external ear canal was markedly erythematous and several ulcerations were present along the vertical and horizontal canal walls. A moderate amount of purulent debris was present in the canal and the tympanic membrane appeared to be intact.

i. Cytology of the exudate is shown (56). What are the differential diagnoses for this patient?

ii. Culture and susceptibility isolated solely *Aspergillus niger* from the ear. What is the pathogenesis of this condition with regard to this specific patient?

57 The Chinese shar pei dog is phenotypically identified as having 'excessive folds and wrinkles'.

i. What metabolic disease is this breed predisposed to as a result of the genetic mutation that causes the excessive wrinkling (57)?

ii. What disease in people is clinically similar?

iii. How is this disease treated?

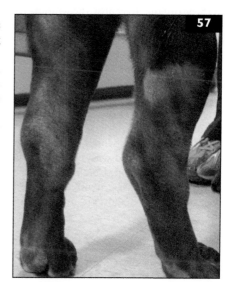

56 i. Cytology shows neutrophilic exudate with ceruminous debris. Septate hyphae are also present. Otomycosis would be the top differential. Secondary bacterial otitis externa cannot be ruled out despite the lack of bacterial organisms detected on cytology.
ii. *Aspergillus* spp. are found in the environment in soil and organic debris. They produce small (2–3 µm) airborne conidia, which land on animate and inanimate objects. In most cases, these organisms represent transient inhabitants of the skin and hair in healthy individuals; however, *Aspergillus* can produce opportunistic infection in compromised individuals through mucosal or cutaneous surfaces. Nasal aspergillosis is the most common presentation in dogs. Cutaneous lesions are noted with disseminated disease and are rarely seen in healthy animals. This may be accompanied by musculoskeletal changes, neurologic signs, respiratory disease, or gastrointestinal illness. German shepherd dogs, particularly young to middle-aged females, are overrepresented, suggesting a possible inherited immunologic defect. In a recent literature review, cases of otomycosis due to *Aspergillus* spp. were evaluated. Compromised aural health is suspected to be involved in disease pathogenesis. With regard to this dog, both the history of previous episodes of otitis externa as well as the noted immunocompromised state may have led to the development of otomycosis.

57 i. Familial shar pei fever (FSF). It is estimated that 23% of shar pei dogs are affected by this autoinflammatory disease. FSF is characterized by chronic recurrent episodes of high fever and inflammation of the joints (especially tibiotarsal joints). Episodes can occur every few weeks or months. Secondary complications of the disease are reactive amyloidosis and kidney or liver failure due to amyloid deposits in these organs. Recently, the genome of Chinese shar pei dogs was compared with that of other dogs; a unique 16.1 Kb duplication was identified on the gene that codes for production of an important rate-limiting enzyme (HAS2) in hyaluronan synthesis. This is believed to be the causative mutation for both excessive hyaluronanosis and FSF.
ii. Familial Mediterranean fever. The finding that HAS2 is associated with FSF as well as with sterile fever and inflammation is of interest, as this canine disease may offer clues to the etiology of the disease in people and/or be an animal model of the disease.
iii. With colchicine, which is used to prevent excessively high levels of uric acid in the blood associated with episodes of gout. Potential adverse effects include bone marrow suppression. Colchicine binds selectively and reversibly to microtubules, causing metaphase arrest and preventing many cell functions including degranulation, chemotaxis, and mitosis.

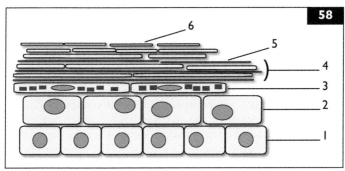

58 A diagrammatic representation of the skin is shown (58).
i. Identify layers 1, 2, 3, 4, 5, and 6.
ii. How does layer 5 form? What are the components of this layer?
iii. What is transepidermal water loss (TEWL)? How is it measured?

59 A 2-year-old female spayed Egyptian Mau cat presented for severe pruritus involving the head, neck, and ear pinnae. According to the owner, who adopted the cat from a rescue organization 6 months prior to presentation, pruritus ranged from moderate to severe and frequently progressed to self-induced excoriation over the cervical region. Scarring was present over the dorsal cervical region due to repeated, severe self-trauma (59). No response to aggres-

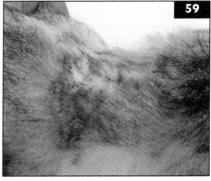

sive parasite control (including an ivermectin treatment trial, lime sulfur dips, and monthly application of adulticide flea prevention) or antimicrobial therapy for bacteria or yeast was reported.
i. What are your differential diagnoses for this patient?
ii. What reaction patterns have been associated with cutaneous reactions to food in the cat?
iii. What does a 'novel protein hypoallergenic diet' consist of?

58 i. 1 = basal cell layer; 2 = spinous cell layer; 3 = granular layer; 4 = corneal layer; 5 = epidermal lipid layer; 6 = cornified cells undergoing desquamation.

ii. The epidermal lipid layer (5) is formed from lamellar granules fusing with the cell membrane at the junction of the granular layer (3) and the corneal layer (4). When lamellar granules fuse with cell membranes and expel their contents into the intercellular space, the contents are modified by enzymes. Glycolipids are converted to ceramides by glucosidases and phospholipids to fatty acids by phospholipases. This results in the formation of the 'barrier lipids', which are comprised of ceramides, cholesterol, and free fatty acids. Ceramides are the dominant lipid and are generated from a sphingoid base and a fatty acid. The sphingoid base includes, but is not limited to, sphingosine, dihydrosphingosine, and phytosphingosine.

iii. TEWL refers to the amount of water vapor lost through the stratum corneum each day. In healthy people this is estimated to be 0.5 liters/day; in people with psoriasis, loss can be as high as 6 liters/day. TEWL is measured with a probe applied to the skin using either a closed or an open chamber. Closed chambered probes are not affected by ambient or body-induced airflows. Open chamber probes can be affected by ambient and body-induced airflows, probe size, and the angle of measurement. Air currents, room temperature, and ambient humidity can also affect test results.

59 i. Allergy (cutaneous adverse reaction to food, environmental allergies), dermatophytosis, injection site reaction, vasculitis, reaction to topical flea control or other topical medication.

ii. Miliary dermatitis, eosinophilic skin lesions (granuloma, plaque, indolent ulcer), erosions/ulcerations of the head and neck (cervical–facial pruritic dermatitis), and self-induced symmetrical alopecia. Compared with other feline allergic skin diseases, cats with food allergy more frequently present with lesions affecting the head, neck, and pinnae.

iii. A protein is considered 'novel' if the animal has not been exposed to the protein even in small quantities. A 'novel protein hypoallergenic diet' may be a home-prepared diet or a limited ingredient commercial diet. Many dermatologists regard the home-prepared novel protein diet to be the 'gold standard' for evaluating food allergy in the dog and cat, as the ingredients and additives are completely controlled. Limited ingredient diets need to be carefully evaluated when used in an elimination diet trial to ensure that other potential allergens (animal by-products, additional protein and/or carbohydrate sources) are not included on the ingredients list. (**Note:** Manufacturing control can be variable; a recent study detected common food allergens in diets often used for elimination diet trials [non-prescription, over-the-counter] even when the ingredients were not listed on the package.)

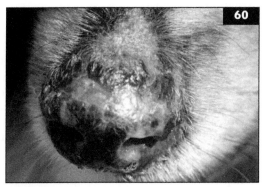

60 A 3-year-old dog presented for a second opinion on the management of these nasal lesions (60).

i. What are the possible differential diagnoses?

ii. The pathologist noted the following key findings: 'lichenoid interface dermatitis with basal cell degeneration and apoptosis, no signs of inflammatory cells in the cutaneous or follicular epidermal layers, and pigmentary incontinence'. What is the most compatible diagnosis?

iii. What are the treatment options for this disease?

61 What common pitfalls are associated with diagnosing food allergy in dogs or cats?

60 i. Lupus erythematosus, mucocutaneous pyoderma, dermatophytosis, pemphigus, *Malassezia* overgrowth, vitiligo, trauma, cutaneous lymphoma, uveodermatologic syndrome.

ii. Lupus erythematosus.

iii. In severe cases, remission needs to be induced with aggressive prednisone/prednisolone therapy (2–4 mg/kg PO divided q12h). Once remission is achieved, long-term care requires a second immunosuppressive agent as the steroid dose is gradually decreased (over months). One option is cyclosporine (5 mg/kg PO q24h); once in remission it may be possible to reduce the dose. Intermittent waxing and waning of lesions can occur. Potent topical steroids or tacrolimus can be used as adjunct therapy. In mild cases, oral combinations can be used as initial therapy in place of steroids, and adjunct topical steroids or tacrolimus used at the beginning of therapy or for relapses. Topical treatment of the nose is difficult and complications include mechanical removal, difficulty finding a potent topical steroid in a penetrating base, continued client compliance, thinning of the nasal planum, secondary nasal cartilage erosion, arteriole hemorrhage, and elevations in liver enzymes, as topical steroids are absorbed systemically. Owners should wear gloves when applying topical therapies to the nose.

61 Include, but are not limited to: not feeding the diet long enough to fully evaluate a response; failure to select a 'novel' protein based on the animal's previous dietary history (including consideration of potentially cross-reactive food allergens [e.g. cross-reaction of other feathered poultry such as goose, turkey, or duck with chicken; cross-reaction of bison with beef]); reaction of the animal to the hydrolyzed diet when allergy to parent protein is present; failing to control secondary pruritic skin disease (e.g. external parasites, secondary bacterial pyoderma, or *Malassezia* overgrowth); failure of the diet trial to be completely strict. Exclusion of flavored medications (particularly parasite prevention, certain antibiotics, NSAIDs), animal-based chew toys (rawhide, pigs' ears, 'bully bones'), normal treats, table scraps, food used to hide medication, and gelatin-containing products or medications (certain marshmallows, medication capsules) is necessary.

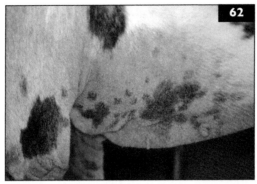

62 A three-year-old male neutered Great Dane dog (68 kg [150 lb]) presented because of lack of response to immunotherapy. The dog had been diagnosed with AD two years ago via IDT and has been receiving ASIT for months. Other than immunotherapy, the dog is not currently receiving any other medication, but review of the medical records reveals numerous courses of antibiotics including cefpodoxime (200 mg/day) and enrofloxacin (2.5 mg/kg). Representative clinical signs of the dermatologic examination are shown (62). Other than the skin, physical examination is normal. Dermatologic examination reveals extensive superficial pyoderma on the ventral abdomen, diffuse lichenification, and thickening of the skin on the ventrum, in flexor areas, medial aspects of the legs, ventral neck, and ears. There is a diffuse papular eruption on the dog's ventrum. The dog's coat is 'greasy' and malodorous. The dog's vaccinations are current and the owners have administered inconsistent flea and tick control. Skin scrapings for demodicosis were negative. Skin cytology revealed large numbers of *Malassezia* organisms, cocci, and neutrophils. A bacterial culture isolated an oxacillin-resistant SIG susceptible only to chloramphenicol.
i. The owners believe that the immunotherapy has failed. What is your response?
ii. What is your treatment plan for this dog at this time?
iii. The dog returns for a recheck visit 6 weeks later. What will be your plan if the dog is severely pruritic, moderately pruritic, or not pruritic at all?

63 What are probiotics? What skin diseases may benefit from their use?

62 i. It is impossible to assess accurately the dog's response to immunotherapy; inconsistent flea prevention (possible flare factor) and secondary microbial infections may be masking true efficacy of ASIT.

ii. Restart flea control and aggressively treat the microbial overgrowth before pursuing further diagnostics. The dog should be bathed at least 2–3 times a week in medicated shampoo; a combination antibacterial/antifungal shampoo should be used. If the dog cannot be bathed frequently, a thorough sprayed application of 2% chlorhexidine solution can substitute for one bath. Systemic ketoconazole (5 mg/kg q24h) in addition to topical antifungal shampoo therapy is beneficial. Oral antibiotic treatment for bacterial pyoderma is difficult, as the only drug available for use is chloramphenicol. Although effective, the drug requires three times daily administration and can cause nausea and vomiting. Owners need to wear gloves when administering the drug and when cleaning up any vomitus; aplastic anemia is a risk in people.

iii. If the dog is severely pruritic at recheck and microbial overgrowth has resolved, response to a treatment trial for scabies should be discussed with the clients. If the dog is non-pruritic, one assumption is that the intense pruritus was due to the combined bacterial/yeast infection. Given the strength of IDT and clinical history, continued ASIT would be advisable. If the dog is improved but still pruritic, a food trial would be indicated. If that fails to resolve the problem, before repeating IDT, owner compliance with therapy should be assessed, again.

63 A 'probiotic' is defined as 'live microorganisms which, when administered in adequate amounts, confer a health benefit to the host'. The most commonly used probiotics are strains of lactic acid fermenting bacteria such as *Lactobacillus*, *Bifidobacterium*, and *Streptococcus* (*S. thermophilus*). Their mechanism of action is not well understood, but three major modes of action have been suggested: probiotics might be able to modulate the host's defenses including the innate as well as the acquired immune system; probiotics may have a direct effect on other microorganisms (commensal and/or pathogenic ones); probiotic effects may be based on actions affecting microbial products such as toxins. Probiotic use has been studied in a wide range of diseases, but small pilot studies have suggested that their administration may protect against allergies.

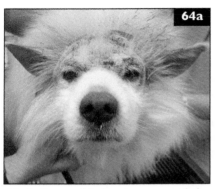
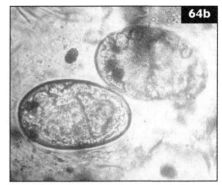

64 A 7-year-old dog is presented for the problem of crusting and scaling of 2 months' duration (64a). Past pertinent history includes a diagnosis of cutaneous lymphoma in the last year; the dog was in remission at the time of presentation. The owners report that the dog is not pruritic. Skin scrapings were negative for *Demodex* mites, but large numbers of oval eggs were found on skin scraping (64b).
i. What are these organisms?
ii. What is the diagnosis, and how does it relate to the dog's past pertinent history?
iii. How would you treat this dog?

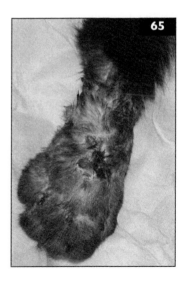

65 A 7-year-old male castrated DSH cat is presented for the lesions shown (65). Only a single limb is affected on examination. Both the dorsal and ventral surfaces of the distal limb have multiple cutaneous nodules and draining tracts. The cat is noted to be indoor/outdoor and will frequently stay out overnight. No known trauma predisposed the lesion development; however, the owner is not sure what happens with the cat on nights he stays away from home. The cat is otherwise healthy, is not currently being administered any medications other than monthly topical parasite preventive, and is up to date on vaccinations.
i. Given the nodular clinical appearance of the lesions, what are your differential diagnoses?
ii. What diagnostic tests are recommended?

Answers: 64, 65

64 i. *Sarcoptes scabiei* mite eggs.

ii. Sarcoptes infestation or scabies is highly contagious and a known zoonosis. There are two atypical presentations in dogs. The first is scabies incognito. Dogs are intensely pruritic, there may be a mild eosinophilia, but classic lesions are absent. The second presentation is 'crusted scabies', or what was once called 'Norwegian' scabies, because it was first recognized in Norway in 1848 in a group of people with leprosy. In crusted scabies, immunosuppression from drugs (corticosteroids, anti-neoplastic drugs) allows for rapid proliferation of mites with little host immune response. Classically, these dogs have little to no pruritus and a thick gray scaly material that contains large numbers of mites.

iii. All in-contact dogs require treatment. The dog will require bathing to remove the thick crusts containing mites and debris. Preventive parasite control is important adjunct therapy in patients being treated for chronic medical diseases (e.g. neoplasia). Effective systemic therapies for scabies include: selamectin (6–12 mg/kg every 2 weeks for 4 treatments); ivermectin (0.2–0.4 mg/kg PO every 7 days for 4–6 weeks); doramectin (0.2–0.6 mg/kg SC every 7 days for 4–6 weeks); milbemycin (0.5–2.0 mg/kg PO q24h for 30 days). Effective topical therapies include amitraz (every 2 weeks for 6 weeks), fipronil spray (3–6 ml applied as a sponge-on weekly for 4–6 weeks), and lime sulfur (every 5 days for 6 weeks).

65 i. Include infectious (bacterial deep pyoderma including atypical bacteria such as *Nocardia*, *Actinomyces*, *Mycobacterium* spp.; deep fungal infection, including blastomycosis, cryptococcosis, histoplasmosis, sporotrichosis, opportunistic fungal infection), inflammatory (sterile pyogranuloma/granuloma syndrome, histiocytic disease), or neoplasia (squamous cell carcinoma, soft tissue sarcoma). Foreign body reaction or trauma with secondary infection should also be considered for this patient.

ii. Cytology of the exudates and culture and susceptibility looking for bacterial and fungal infections. Because of the inherent danger of culturing deep fungal organisms and zoonotic transmission, unstained cytologic preparations should be included with the culture specimen. The laboratory can stain these and possibly identify an infectious agent. Biopsy of the nodules is recommended to confirm the diagnosis. Radiographs and/or advanced imaging of the limb may be indicated if other diagnostics fail to identify an underlying cause for the lesions. A fistulogram to identify draining tracts can be helpful when foreign body reaction is present. In this case, skin biopsy revealed branching pigmented fungi on special stains; a diagnosis of phaeohyphomycosis was made. This organism was most likely inoculated via a puncture wound. Definitive diagnosis requires submission of a wedge of tissue to a diagnostic laboratory familiar with advanced fungal culture techniques. Surgical excision is often the treatment of choice.

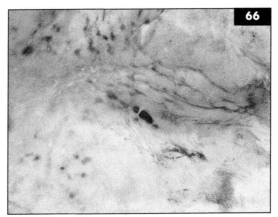

66 A 6-year-old, indoor/outdoor FeLV/FIV-negative intact male cat developed soft tissue abscessation as shown (66). Despite repeated lancing, draining, and flushing procedures with concomitant courses of cefovecin injections and oral amoxicillin over the past 2 months, the lesions fail to heal. Other than these draining nodular skin lesions, which appear to be limited to the inguinal fat pad, the cat is apparently in good health.
i. Name the 'dermatologic problem' along with differential diagnoses that should be excluded.
ii. What diagnostic tests are indicated?
iii. Pending a diagnosis, what treatment might be considered?

67 i. What is a hydrolyzed hypoallergenic diet?
ii. What evidence is available to support or refute the use of hydrolyzed diets in suspected allergic patients?

66 i. 'Non-healing panniculitis' restricted to the inguinal fat pad. Differential diagnoses include: inflammatory/infectious (deep methicillin-resistant staphylococcal pyoderma, nocardiosis, actinomycosis, L-form bacteriosis, rapidly-growing mycobacteriosis [RGM], subcutaneous mycoses), inflammatory/non-infectious (foreign body, sterile panniculitis), and possibly neoplasia.

ii. Diagnostic imaging to determine the extent of the lesions and whether or not a foreign body is present. Surgical exploration of inguinal skin with aseptic procurement of deep subcutaneous wedges for culture and biopsy is required. Punch biopsy specimens of nodules will not get deep tissue and may not provide the laboratory with enough tissue for culture since organisms may be present in small quantities (especially rapidly-growing *Mycobacteria* spp.). As some organisms in the differential list are better seen cytologically, fine-needle aspirates of intact deep nodules and/or direct impressions of cut sections of deep tissue can be made and submitted.

iii. Doxycycline could be administered for presumptive RGM. Selection of this antibiotic would also target L-form bacteria as its mechanism of action is independent of the presence of a bacterial cell wall. This cat had RGM, as evidenced by few aggregates of acid-fast bacilli within nodular pyogranulomatous inflammation of the panniculus.

67 i. A parent protein (typically chicken or soy) is broken into smaller amino acid fragments, which are then incorporated into the diet. Hydrolyzed diets are formulated through enzymatic degradation and ultrafiltration to remove large molecules and higher molecular weight peptides.

ii. In people, food allergy is a type 1 hypersensitivity reaction caused by binding of epitopes or proteins to IgE molecules. These large molecules (>10 kDa) cross-link IgE molecules on the surface of mast cells, leading to degranulation. Of food allergens identified in the dog, allergenic proteins all had a molecular weight of >20 kDa. Depending on the degree of hydrolysis, the molecule size of hydrolyzed dietary amino acids ranges from <3 kDa (extensively hydrolyzed) to 10 kDa (partially hydrolyzed). In an infant cow's milk allergy study, it was noted that the smaller molecule size was not able to cause IgE cross-linking, thereby preventing an allergic reaction from occurring. The pathogenesis of food allergy in veterinary species is not fully elucidated; however, cutaneous type 1 reactions have been noted both immediately and later with food exposure in dogs and cats. Both immunologic and non-immunologic cutaneous adverse reactions to food exist. A systematic review uncovered evidence that suggests reduced immunologic and clinical allergenicity of hydrolyzed diets in dogs with food allergy. Some dogs, however, experienced recurrence of allergic symptoms when fed hydrolyzed diets; this was true in dogs with food allergy of undetermined origin and in dogs with confirmed food allergy to the parent protein used in the hydrolyzed diet. Whether this is true in cats with food allergy is not known.

68 The diagnosis of AD is based on the exclusion of all other causes of pruritic skin disease. It relies on the patient's signalment, past pertinent history, and clinical signs. It is widely accepted that there is no test available that will diagnose the disease; 'allergy tests' are used once the clinical diagnosis has been made to support the clinician's diagnosis, to document IgE involvement (i.e. rule out atopic-like dermatitis), and to help guide immunotherapy formulation if this is to be used as part of the disease management.

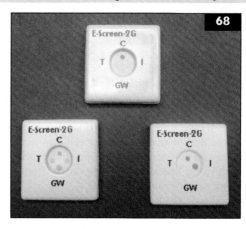

i. What are the two categories of 'allergy tests' available?
ii. What is the principle behind the use of these tests in allergic disease?
iii. What is shown (**68**)?

69 A 9-year-old female spayed keeshond dog was presented for multiple deeply pigmented plaque-like lesions on the ventral abdomen (**69**). The owner reported that the plaques had been present for several years, appeared to wax and wane (exfoliate and regress), but always recurred at the same site. There was no evidence that the lesions were bothersome to the dog, but the owner was concerned about possible neoplasia.

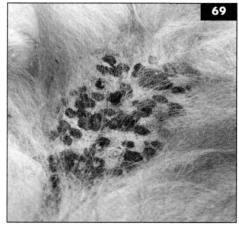

i. What is the most likely diagnosis?
ii. What is the presumed underlying etiology?
iii. With regard to prognosis, what do you tell the owner?

68 i. Allergen-specific IgE serology, intradermal allergy tests.

ii. Allergen-specific IgE serology tests detect circulating IgE antibody in serum directed against a panel of environmental allergens. Most are ELISA-based tests (others use radioallergosorbent tests); patient serum is added to allergen extracts (in liquid or solid phase) and reaction is determined by antigen–antibody binding. This is detected either by colorimetric, fluorometric, or radiometric analysis. Intradermal testing also demonstrates IgE-mediated allergen hypersensitivity by intradermal injections of various environmental allergens. Allergens bind to IgE molecules on sensitized mast cells, causing degranulation; this leads to localized extravasation of edema fluid, erythema, and formation of a wheal. 'Positive results' with either test are interpreted with regard to 'importance' based on the patient's history and seasonality.

iii. Allercept® E-screen, second generation, available only in European countries (not USA). This rapid screening immunoassay allergy test incorporates the same principles of complete serum-based allergen panels (ELISA-based technology utilizing highly specific IgE detection reagent). Mixtures of allergens from environmental groups (trees, grasses/weeds, indoor allergens) are 'spotted' onto the test cassette to identify positive reactions to the patient's serum by color indicator. This test has been evaluated in dogs and cats for its ability to 'predict' results of a complete serum allergen panel; the test demonstrated good predictability in both species.

69 i. Canine pigmented viral plaques.

ii. The plaques are caused by a papillomavirus that is distinctly different from the virus that causes oral papillomatosis in the dog (canine oral papillomavirus; COPV). At least three strains (COPV3, COPV4, COPV5) have been isolated from pigmented viral plaque lesions in dogs.

iii. There appears to be a genetic predisposition of certain breeds (pug, miniature schnauzer) to develop pigmented viral plaques, although the lesions have been reported in several other breeds. SCC at the site of these lesions has been reported due to transformation of pigmented viral plaques; however, pigmented viral plaques and SCC have been reported on the same animal, making it difficult to be certain about transformation of lesions. The metastatic potential of the lesions in dogs is unknown. In pug dogs, malignant transformation of pigmented viral plaques has not been reported, which differs from other breeds. Recommendations are for owners to monitor lesions. Often, the pigmented plaques will enlarge to a certain point and from there become stable with respect to size. Lesions rarely cause clinical problems for the dog and are mostly cosmetic abnormalities; however, because of the potential for malignant transformation, any change in the lesion should be reported and investigated. Skin biopsy/surgical removal of the lesion would be indicated.

70 i. Are there any drawbacks to the different kinds of 'allergy tests'?
ii. In relation to allergy testing, what significance does 'high-affinity Fc-epsilon receptor' have?

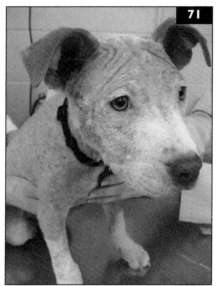

71 A 4-month-old male intact pit bull dog presents for progressive hair loss, pruritus, and a generalized 'rash' on the body. The owner had initially found him as a stray on the side of the road. Shortly after he was adopted, the puppy developed juvenile cellulitis ('puppy strangles'), which was treated with antibiotics and corticosteroid administration. He was still being treated for the juvenile cellulitis at the time of presentation for these problems. His peripheral lymph nodes are still somewhat enlarged on palpation; however, he seems otherwise to be an active and happy puppy. On physical examination you note complete alopecia with areas of 'peach fuzz', widespread erythema, and a severe papular–pustular eruption over the entire body (**71**). All four paws and the face do not have this eruption, but they are erythematous and partially alopecic. You perform multiple deep skin scrapings and note numerous *Demodex canis* mites. Most of the mites are alive and all life stages are present.
i. What are possible reasons for the development of generalized demodicosis?
ii. What are some potential complications of treatment in this patient?

70 i. Serum-based allergy tests have variability between laboratory reagents, protocol, and interpretation methods. Allergenic extracts are one source of variability, which can make test interpretation different between laboratories and between allergen batches. The ability to bind IgE exclusively (as opposed to cross-reacting with IgG) depends on the reagent used; some laboratories use less specific binding reagents, leading to more false-positive reactions. Standardization of protocols and reporting of results vary among laboratories. Sensitivity (44–100%) and specificity (0–100%) is variable for serum-based allergy tests. Allergen extracts also affect intradermal allergy testing. Individual interpretation of reactions is another variable. Variability between individuals is noted with regard to allergens used in testing as well as dilutions. Drug interactions have more influence with intradermal testing than with serum allergy testing. Antihistamines, tricyclic antidepressants, and glucocorticoids require adequate withdrawal to prevent false-negative reactions. Sedation protocols can influence test results; opioids (particularly oxymorphone), ketamine/diazepam, acepromazine, and propofol can all adversely affect results.

ii. It refers to the technique in serum allergy testing in which the assay detects allergen-specific IgE. Reagents bind strongly to the Fc-epsilon receptor, which resides on the alpha chain of IgE molecules. Binding affinity is very high for this receptor; tests that utilize this receptor technology have more specific binding with less cross-reaction and binding of IgG.

71 i. The treatment for juvenile cellulitis may have influenced the development of generalized demodicosis in this patient. As the treatment involves high doses of corticosteroids (high anti-inflammatory to low immunosuppressive doses; 1–2 mg/kg/day) this may have suppressed the puppy's developing immune system, making it more likely for demodicosis to develop. Also, this is a pit bull dog. This breed has been shown to have a higher risk of demodicosis as well as a short hair coat, which may also be a risk factor for this parasitic skin disease.

ii. Since the dog's lymph nodes are persistently enlarged, treatment for juvenile cellulitis is still indicated. Discontinuing treatment prematurely can lead to disease relapse. However, the concurrent corticosteroid administration may make it more difficult to resolve generalized demodicosis. Until the dose can be tapered and discontinued, it is unlikely the demodicosis can be completely cured. Typically, treatment for juvenile cellulitis is discontinued after a few weeks to months. Additionally, dosing for whatever treatment option is elected for generalized demodicosis (e.g. ivermectin, milbemycin oxime, amitraz, moxidectin) will need to be continuously evaluated as the puppy continues to grow and gain weight.

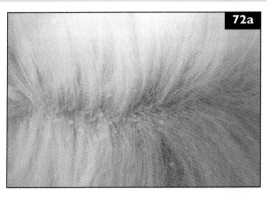

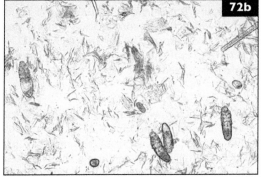

72 A 12-year-old female spayed ragdoll cat presented for generalized excessive scaling and mild pruritus (72a). The cat was also reported to be more lethargic than usual.
i. What are the differential diagnoses for this patient?
ii. This parasite (72b) was identified on skin scraping. What is the definitive diagnosis?
iii. What is the recommended treatment(s) for this condition?

73 With regard to the puppy described in case 71:
i. What is the treatment goal for resolving juvenile-onset generalized demodicosis?
ii. With regard to long-term prognosis, how likely are you to 'cure' this patient?

72 i. Demodicosis, cheyletiellosis, dermatophytosis, bacterial pyoderma, metabolic disease (kidney insufficiency, liver disease), endocrine disease (diabetes mellitus, hyperthyroidism), neoplasia (either primary cutaneous neoplasia [e.g. cutaneous lymphoma] or paraneoplastic syndrome), inability to groom appropriately (obesity, musculoskeletal pain/arthritis).
ii. *Demodex gatoi* infestation.
iii. Based on an evidence-based review of demodicosis treatment protocols, there is evidence to support application of lime sulfur 2% as a topical dip once weekly. As this mite can be rather difficult to find on skin scraping, a lime sulfur trial is recommended to rule out this parasite when suspected. To date, lime sulfur has been the most efficacious treatment for feline *D. gatoi* infestation. There is evidence to support the recommendation of amitraz rinses (0.0125–0.025% weekly). Cats may be more sensitive to side-effects of this treatment option compared with dogs; if considered, it is generally recommended to use a lower concentration. There are anecdotal reports of efficacy of a combination spot-on product containing imidacloprid 10% plus moxidectin 2.5% for treatment of *D. gatoi* infestation; well-designed clinical trials to evaluate this treatment option need to be performed. All in-contact animals (cats) need to be treated as this is considered to be a contagious parasite.

73 i. To achieve 2–3 consecutive negative skin scrapings performed 2–4 weeks apart. A negative skin scrape implies no mites of any life stage identified, alive or dead. Skin scrapings should be performed from the same body region each time to assess treatment efficacy. Treatment for demodicosis should be continued until this end point is reached; premature discontinuation will cause a relapse. On average, this takes several months (7 months on average and sometimes longer); however, the prognosis for resolution is good.
ii. In general, the prognosis is good. Approximately 80% of cases will be cured once the end point of treatment is reached (2–3 consecutive negative skin scrapes, remaining negative on skin scrapes for a full year following treatment discontinuation). The other 20% will have chronic demodicosis; however, these dogs can have a good quality of life and be lesion-free with administration of maintenance miticide therapy. Owners should be educated that although this is an immunologic problem (cell-mediated immunodeficiency in identifying the mites as 'foreign'), it is not a general immunodeficiency; dogs with juvenile-onset demodicosis are no more likely than the average to develop other illness in the future.

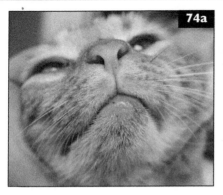

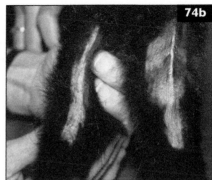

74 What is the clinical diagnosis of each of the images shown (74a–c)? All the cats are otherwise healthy. (a) Firm, painless mass on the chin of a cat. (b) Firm raised symmetrical, hairless, non-pruritic lesions on the caudal thigh of a cat. (c) Lip lesion on a cat.

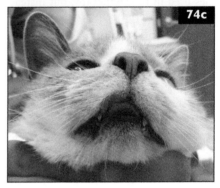

75 Radiation therapy can be a beneficial treatment option for several cutaneous abnormalities. Although it is used most commonly for neoplastic conditions (e.g. mast cell tumor, soft tissue sarcomas), other more 'benign' conditions (e.g. refractory acral lick lesions or eosinophilic granulomas) may also show beneficial responses to radiation therapy.
i. What types of radiation delivery techniques exist in veterinary medicine?
ii. What types of radiation delivery systems exist in veterinary medicine? What are the pros and cons of the options available?

74 These three clinical presentations are part of the 'eosinophilic' reaction pattern of cats. 74a and 74b are 'eosinophilic granuloma' lesions. Their biopsy specimens have acellular foci of eosinophilic granulation around collagen fibers. True collagen fiber degeneration or 'collagenolysis', as evidenced by Masson's trichrome stain, is not a consistent feature of feline eosinophilic granuloma. 74c is a feline indolent ulcer. These lesions may be unilateral or bilateral. Unilateral lesions have been observed to develop at the site of injuries (cacti thorn, tick bite) or infection (*M. canis* infected hair).

75 i. (1) Brachytherapy: a radioactive material is implanted within the treatment area of interest and radiation emanates from inside the patient outwards. (2) Plesiotherapy (contact radiotherapy): utilizes radioactive materials similar to the ones used in brachytherapy, but instead of implanting them within the treatment area, the material is placed on top of the area using a special applicator. (3) Teletherapy (most common delivery technique in veterinary medicine): utilizes either man-made radiation in the form of x-rays or naturally produced gamma rays from decaying radioactive materials.

ii. Linear accelerators and cobalt units. Linear accelerators are machines that accelerate charged particles (typically electrons) using electromagnetic fields. Different x-ray photons and electron beam energies are produced, allowing for the treatment of deep and superficial tumors. Because of their increased flexibility in design and dose delivery, linear accelerators have become the most common delivery system in treatment centers. Unlike linear accelerators, cobalt units are mechanically simple. The radioactive cobalt-60 source emits high-energy radiation in the form of gamma rays as part of the natural decay process. While linear accelerators allow the option to choose which energy photons (for deep-seated tumors) or electrons (for superficial tumors) to use, cobalt units are limited to photons of one energy only and have no electron capability. Since the source is constantly decaying, care is necessary on a daily basis to ensure the safety of the patients and staff who interact with it. With a half-life of about 5.25 years, to maintain adequate output and minimize prolonged treatment times, the source is typically replaced every 5–10 years.

76 A 2-year-old Boston terrier dog presented for non-inflammatory hair loss along the ventral trunk and caudomedial thighs (76). Alopecia had been slow to develop, but was progressively worsening. Skin scrapings and fungal culture were both negative.

i. What is the most likely cause for the alopecia? Describe four syndromes of this condition.

ii. What is tardive alopecia?

iii. If you were to biopsy the skin of this dog, what findings would be compatible with your working diagnosis?

iv. Is there an effective treatment for this condition?

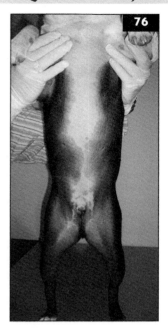

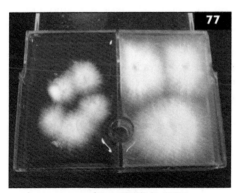

77 **i.** What is dermatophyte test medium (DTM) (77)?

ii. What is the principle of its use, and what is the most common error made when using DTM?

76 i. Pattern alopecia has four recognizable clinical syndromes. The first is pinnal alopecia, most often seen in dachshund dogs. The second syndrome occurs in young American water spaniels and Portuguese water dogs and is characterized as hypotrichosis of the ventral neck, caudomedial thighs, and tail. Syndrome three is typified by greyhound dogs with caudal thigh alopecia. This syndrome is different from bald thigh syndrome (i.e. alopecia of the lateral thigh). The fourth syndrome (this case) is the most common syndrome seen in Boston terriers, dachshunds, Chihuahuas, Manchester terriers, whippets, and greyhound dogs. Beginning at about 6 months of age, these dogs lose hair along the post-auricular area, ventral neck, ventral trunk, and caudomedial thighs.
ii. Localized, regionalized, or generalized hair loss as an animal matures. These animals are born with a normal coat, but alopecia becomes evident as the animal ages. It is assumed that tardive alopecia is an inherited disorder.
iii. Pattern alopecia of dogs is characterized histopathologically by miniaturized hair follicles and hair shafts with normal adnexal structures. The follicles are thin and short, the hair bulbs are smaller than usual, and the hair shafts are fine and thin.
iv. No. In some instances, melatonin orally (3–9 mg/dog q8h) or by subcutaneous implant (usually requires several [8, 12, or 18 mg, based on patient's body weight]) will result in hair growth. If melatonin is effective, new hair growth should be expected within 2 months. Since this condition, with its many clinical forms, is often considered a cosmetic disorder, no treatment is required.

77 i. DTM was first described in 1969 and was developed to aid medics in Vietnam in the identification of griseofulvin-sensitive dermatophytes in soldiers with *Trichophyton* spp. infections. The base is a Sabouraud's dextrose agar with cyclohexamide and antibiotics (gentamicin and chlortetracycline) added to inhibit growth of saprophytic fungi and bacteria. A pH indicator (phenol red) is added to the medium; as dermatophytes grow they produce alkaline metabolites and turn the DTM from yellow (pH 5.5) to red.
ii. Potential dermatophytes will grow faster and create a color change sooner than other saprophytic fungi. The most common problem is the high number of false-positive results when identification of a dermatophyte is made using the red color change as the sole diagnostic criterion. Although all dermatophytes induce a color change, many non-dermatophyte species will induce an almost equally intense color changes. The most common non-pathogenic organisms that can mimic dermatophytes include *Alternaria* spp., *Aspergillus* spp., *Chrysosporium* spp., *Penicillium* spp., and *Scopulariopsis* spp. Many of these saprophytes have similar colony morphology to that of dermatophytes, making microscopic identification mandatory.

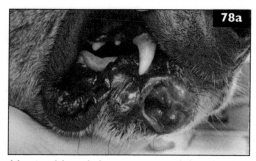

78 A 4-year-old mixed-breed dog is presented for this lesion on its face (78a). The lesion is painful, malodorous, and developed rapidly over 2 weeks. The lesion is firm, movable in the dermis, and does not appear to be attached to underlying tissue. This is the only abnormality found on examination.
i. What are possible differential diagnoses for this mass? What diagnostic tests are indicated?
ii. The biopsy report shows the following: ulceration, perivascular inflammation, severe diffuse infiltrate of eosinophils with large numbers oriented around individual collagen fibers, prominent flame follicles and macrophages and giant cells. There was no growth on bacterial culture and FNA was inflammatory with large numbers of eosinophils and fewer mast cells. What is the diagnosis?

79 A 1-year-old male neutered Labrador retriever dog is shown (79). The owners adopted the dog from a rescue organization and are presenting the dog for a physical examination. The dog was surrendered by the previous owners because they were unable to train the dog to urinate or defecate outside. Physical examination revealed an inactive dog, mental dullness, large broad head, short neck, short limbs, and abnormal dentition. What is the most likely diagnosis?

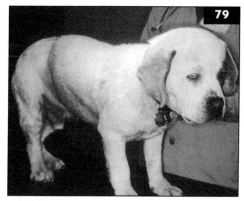

78 i. Tumor, infection, granuloma. Mast cell tumor would be a major differential diagnosis. FNA, multiple impression smears (send several to reference laboratory unstained), deep wedge biopsy, and culture of the lesions. Regarding skin biopsy, in order to obtain a diagnostic specimen, a wedge of tissue should be collected with every effort made to get a deep specimen. Many microbial organisms causing granulomatous lesions create significant inflammation and are only isolated from deep within the lesion. The laboratory should be made aware that potentially zoonotic organisms (e.g. deep fungal mycoses) are a considered differential. Biopsy is the most useful diagnostic test once mast cell tumor is ruled out.

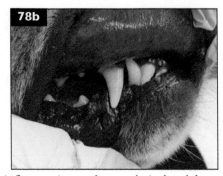

ii. Canine eosinophilic granuloma, an uncommon skin lesion in dogs compared with cats. Typically, lesions are found on the skin, oral cavity, or external ear. The etiology is unknown; hypersensitivity reaction (e.g. arthropod bites) is suspected based on observations that lesions are solitary, do not recur after treatment, and are often found in areas where insect bites tend to occur. Siberian huskies and Cavalier King Charles spaniels are predisposed. Lesions can be successfully treated via excision, but they are usually glucocorticoid responsive. The lesion responded completely to three subcutaneous injections of methylprednisolone without reported recurrence (78b).

79 Congenital hypothyroidism or cretinism. This occurs when there is absent or ineffective TSH, dyshormonogenesis of thyroid hormone, or defects in thyroid gland development. If pituitary function is normal, the failure of thyroid hormone production results in a goiter. In most cases of canine congenital hypothyroidism, goiters are absent. Congenital hypothyroidism has been reported in several breeds of dogs. In toy fox terriers and rat terriers, a nonsense mutation in the thyroperoxidase gene causing hypothyroidism with goiter has been reported. A lack of production of TSH is the suspected cause of juvenile hypothyroidism in giant schnauzer, boxer, and Scottish deerhound breed dogs.

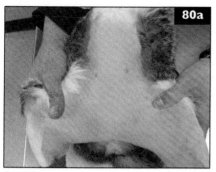

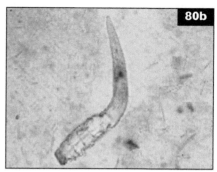

80 This 12-year-old indoor only female spayed DSH cat presented for self-induced alopecia of the ventral abdomen. The cat had a previous diagnosis of allergic skin disease and this was managed with intermittent long-acting injectable corticosteroids for several years. Recently, however, the cat had been losing more hair (80a). The owner also noted that the cat had been gaining weight and had been urinating more frequently; the owner reported that the litter box is 'wetter than normal'. Although there is little in the history and clinical signs suggestive of dermatophytosis, the owner insisted on a fungal culture being performed prior to allowing any further diagnostics because of the cat having ringworm as a kitten. A skin scraping was performed from the cat's abdomen (80b).

i. What is this organism?
ii. What is the difference between this skin disease in cats versus dogs?
iii. How is the condition managed?

81 When it comes to evaluating the outcome of clinical trials, it can be difficult to determine objectively how much a certain therapeutic intervention is or is not helping with regard to disease control. This can be particularly difficult in diseases with a highly variable clinical appearance and severity, such as AD. Because of this, various scales have been developed to help standardize measurements to allow for comparisons between various clinical trial outcomes.

i. What is CADESI?
ii. What is a Visual Analog Scale?

80 i. *Demodex cati.*

ii. Two *Demodex* spp. mites are found in cats: *D. cati* and *D. gatoi. D. gatoi* is considered to be contagious and typically is noted with moderate to severe pruritus. With *D. cati* infestation, identification of this mite should strongly raise concerns about underlying systemic illness. It is often reported in association with FeLV and FIV, diabetes mellitus, hyperadrenocorticism, and neoplasia. To date, there is no evidence that cats have a disease process similar to canine juvenile-onset demodicosis.

iii. When *D. cati* mites are identified and an obvious underlying cause (e.g. excessive use of glucocorticoids, neoplasia) is not identified, thorough medical evaluation is indicated. Diagnostics may include CBC, serum biochemistries, urinalysis, retroviral testing, and possibly thoracic radiographs, abdominal ultrasound, or CT. Identification of the concurrent systemic illness and initiation of treatment are a necessary part of the management. If the underlying disease is managed, the demodicosis may resolve on its own. There is no FDA (USA) approved treatment for feline demodicosis. There are no evidence-based studies on the efficacy of compounds for the treatment of feline demodicosis because of the lack of randomized controlled studies. Therefore, at best the treatment recommendations are based on clinical observations. Treatments include lime sulfur, ivermectin, milbemycin, amitraz, fipronil, and, most recently, topical moxidectin/imidacloprid.

81 i. Canine Atopic Dermatitis Extent and Severity Index, a measurement system that evaluates clinical lesion appearance and severity in atopic dogs based on body site affected. It was designed along the same lines as the SCORAD (SCORing Atopic Dermatitis) measurement system, which is used to assess the clinical severity of AD in people. Both systems attempt to 'quantify' the disease as objectively as possible.

ii. A measurement tool often used with owners for determining severity of pruritus in patients with AD. Various forms of the analog scale exist; however, among the different forms, certain features hold constant. The scales are typically in the form of either a vertical or horizontal line with text descriptions of activities indicating pruritus (**81**). The scale may or may not include graduated lines or number rankings between the text descriptions to further subdivide the scale line. Owners are asked to mark on the scale where they feel their pet currently ranks in relation to the descriptive activities.

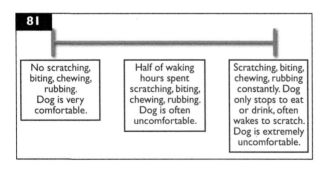

82 A 4-year-old female spayed Cavalier King Charles spaniel dog is presented with a 24-hour history of acute right head tilt and right facial drooping. On physical examination the dog is normal and is bright and interactive. Her neurologic examination is also normal except for a persistent right head tilt, horizontal nystagmus with fast phase towards the left, absent right palpebral reflex, and absent nasal reflex. The nystagmus does not change direction or speed with rotation of the head, but the dog does develop a positional ventrolateral strabismus with extreme dorsoflexion of the head and neck. Based on the examination, what cranial nerves are affected?

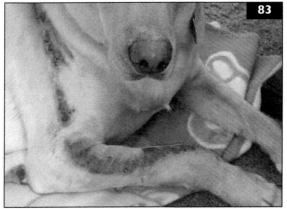

83 A 2-year-old female spayed Labrador retriever dog was presented with a 3-month history of skin lesions. The lesions began as a solitary mass between the shoulders and gradually enlarged to involve the right shoulder, forelimb, and right carpus (83). The lesion was linear and well circumscribed at the time of presentation. The dog was not lame, but the lesions were somewhat pruritic. Skin scrapings and fungal culture were negative, bacterial culture and susceptibility showed no growth, and there was no response to trial antibiotic therapy using cephalexin and fluoroquinolone antibiotics. Impression smears at the time of referral revealed shed keratinocytes, eosinophils, and neutrophils with variable numbers of acantholytic keratinocytes.
i. What are possible differential diagnoses?
ii. Skin biopsy findings revealed subcorneal and intraepidermal eosinophilic and neutrophilic acantholytic pustular dermatitis. What is the diagnosis?

82 The facial nerve (CN7) originates in the rostral medulla, courses out of the brainstem through the internal acoustic meatus, across the petrosal portion of the temporal bone in the facial canal and exits the skull through the stylomastoid foramen. Damage anywhere along the course of the nerve can result in inability to move the lips, eyelids, or nares. To test the facial nerve you need a sensation (transmitted by the trigeminal nerve [CN5]) and a response (performed by the motor nerve [CN7]). **Note:** If either CN5 or CN7 is malfunctioning, these reflexes will be absent. To isolate the trigeminal nerve from the facial nerve, perform a corneal reflex. If the corneal reflex is normal and the palpebral reflex is abnormal, CN7 must be the cause of palpebral reflex failure.

Head tilt, nystagmus, and positional strabismus are indications of vestibular system dysfunction. The vestibulocochlear nerve (CN8) is a sensory nerve; it begins at the receptors in the petrous temporal bone (inner ear) then courses through the internal acoustic meatus, next to the fibers of CN7, to the rostral medulla. Head tilt is the classic symptom of vestibular dysfunction, typically towards the side of the lesion. Abnormal nystagmus occurs when the animal is at rest, and is described by the direction (horizontal, vertical, rotary) and fast phase. The direction of nystagmus is not used to localize to a specific side or anatomic location; it must be interpreted as supportive evidence of vestibular disease. Positional strabismus occurs because of a disruption of coordination between the vestibular system and the nerves that innervate the periocular muscles (CNs 3, 4, 6). Positional strabismus is best visualized with extreme dorsoflexion of the neck. This does not indicate dysfunction in CNs 3, 4, or 6 because the animal has normal eye posture without dorsoflexion. This dog has evidence of right CN7 and 8 dysfunction.

83 i. Nevoid malformation, linear trauma, idiopathic linear pustular acantholytic dermatosis, pemphigus, infectious agent (e.g. sporotrichosis), dermatophytosis, vasculitis, lymphangitis.
ii. Idiopathic linear pustular acantholytic dermatosis. This is a rare disease with unique clinical features including marked linear development of lesions and skin biopsies compatible with pemphigus. To date it has been reported in young dogs and presents as a unilateral lesion. Lesions have been reported to affect the limbs and face. The relationship to pemphigus is unknown in spite of the similarities in lesions associated with the two disease conditions. Dogs may respond completely to glucocorticoid therapy and the occurrence may be a one-time event; other dogs may be refractory to treatment and/or experience multiple relapses and spontaneous remissions.

84 This lesion (84a), located on the proximal dorsal one-third of the tail, is seen in a 5-year-old dog. The owner reports that the mass 'falls off from time to time'. What is the most likely diagnosis?

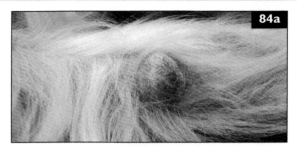

85 A referring veterinarian presented her dog, a 4-year-old male castrated Labrador retriever, with a 2-month history of depigmentation along the upper lip and philtrum. The lesions were multifocal and bordered the haired and non-haired skin; four totally depigmented circular areas were present along the upper muzzle along the border of the lip. As can be seen (85), the lesions were subtle. There

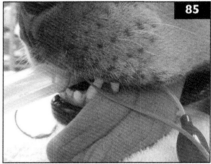

was no evidence that the lesions were causing discomfort; no rubbing, scratching, or rolling was reported. The owner reported having changed food dishes (from plastic to ceramic) at or around the first time lesions were noted; however, new lesions continued to develop.
i. What diagnostics do you recommend for this patient?
ii. What differential diagnoses are you considering?
iii. A biopsy was performed, which showed round cells infiltrating the superficial dermis, epidermis, and multiple hair follicles. Occasionally, small aggregates of round cells were present, forming microabscesses within the epidermis. Immunohistochemistry was strongly positive for CD3. Antigen receptor rearrangement PCR assay revealed a clonal population of T cells. Based on these findings, what is your diagnosis?
iv. Is this a common appearance of the disease?

84b

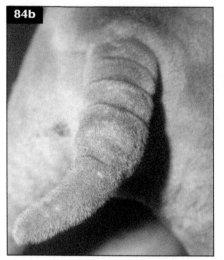

84c

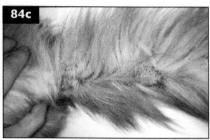

84 The lesion is located in the area of the oval tail gland. This is a concentrated area of sebaceous glands. The history and clinical signs are most compatible with a cutaneous horn or focal area of hyperkeratosis that sloughs off from the tail. This site can be affected by primary disorders of keratinization, focal areas of alopecia (**84b**), or areas of focal infection. Cats have similar collections of sebaceous glands on their tail, but they are present along the entire surface. One manifestation of a primary disorder of keratinization in cats is 'stud tail' (**84c**). Although the name implies this is a disease of intact male cats, lesions can be seen in intact and neutered cats of either sex.

85 i. Skin scraping or hair trichograms to look for *Demodex canis* mites, based on the appearance and location of the lesions. Also cytology to look for overgrowth of bacteria and yeast. A fungal culture is indicated if the dog spends time outside (digging in dirt) or if the history suggests contact with a cat at risk for dermatophytosis. If these tests fail to yield diagnostic information, a skin biopsy is indicated.

ii. Include demodicosis, dermatophytosis, bacterial overgrowth, *Malassezia* overgrowth, possible contact hypersensitivity (although the asymmetrical pattern is a bit unusual for this condition), vitiligo, cutaneous lymphoma, healing wound, foreign body reaction.

iii. Cutaneous epitheliotropic T-cell lymphoma.

iv. This is not a typical appearance to the disease. By the time the patient is presented for examination it is common for the disease to be extensive. This is a very early presentation of cutaneous lymphoma. Many owners would not notice these lesions until they are much more obvious.

86 With regard to radiation therapy:
i. What is the difference between a definitive and a palliative treatment protocol?
ii. What is tomotherapy (86)?

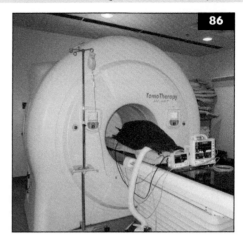

87 A 5-year-old female spayed indoor cat was presented for the problem of chronic grooming of the perianal area. Examination revealed erythema of the anal area and hair loss on the base of the tail. The anal glands were empty on manual expression. The cat was treated with a 21-day course of amoxicillin (10 mg/kg PO q12h) for a presumed anal gland infection. The owners reported continued grooming post treatment; the anal glands were infused with antibiotic steroid cream, which provided temporary relief. Clinical signs, however, returned within 2 weeks. Chronic anal gland inflammation was diagnosed and the anal glands were 'flushed' with an unknown compound. Within 48 hours the cat developed exudation and marked pain and was presented for evaluation. At the time of examination the cat had developed bilateral draining tracts and fecal incontinence (87).

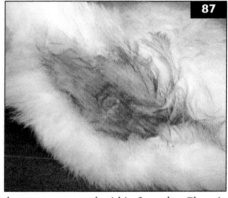

i. The cat is suspected of having an anal gland abscess. What is the most important rule out?
ii. What is the most likely cause of the cat's pruritus?

86 i. Definitive protocols are designed specifically to give the patient the highest probability of a cure or durable control over local/locoregional disease. They are formulated to deliver a larger total dose using many smaller doses (fractions) of radiation over longer periods of total treatment time (weeks). Definitive protocols exchange the acute loss of quality of life (acute toxicities such as desquamation) and a small risk of lifelong morbidities (late toxicities such as skin fibrosis) for the potential of a cure or increase in overall survival. Palliative protocols are designed to give the patient the highest quality of life by addressing a specific clinical sign. They typically are formulated to deliver a smaller total dose using few larger doses of radiation over a variable amount of total treatment time. Palliative treatments exchange treatment-induced morbidity, overall survival, and a larger risk of lifelong morbidities associated with treatment for an immediate improvement in quality of life.

ii. Helical tomotherapy represents hybridization between a linear accelerator and helical CT scanner. Helical tomotherapy encompasses most of the parts of a conventional linear accelerator, but mounts them on a slip ring style gantry. This allows for complex dose distributions that maximize dose to the tumor while minimizing dose to normal structures. Onboard detectors within the system provide CT images of the patient, which provide information for reproducible, fraction-to-fraction repositioning, minimizing the risk of tumor miss or unrecognized high-dose gradients in normal structures. These detectors also provide dose verification and reconstruction, which can help detect and correct variations from the planned dose. For complex target shapes, multiple simultaneous treatment of targets, or advanced stages (size), helical tomotherapy will outperform most linear accelerators available in veterinary medicine.

87 i. Anal gland carcinoma.

ii. Anal gland abscesses and impactions are uncommon in cats. Cats rarely 'scoot' like dogs, but instead will lick and/or traumatize the hairs on the base of their tail. Anal gland inflammation is also uncommon in cats. The lack of response to standard therapy for anal gland infection but response to a locally applied steroid suggests an underlying pruritic cause in this case. The most common allergic skin diseases of cats are flea allergy, AD, and food allergy. In this case, the cat was diagnosed with AD and was well managed with ASIT. The cat underwent surgical removal of the remnant anal gland and necrotic tissue. The area was cleaned regularly and monitored for fecal and urine scalding. Neurologic examination revealed that there was still some sphincter tone and over a 1-year period the cat regained enough sphincter tone to resolve the incontinence.

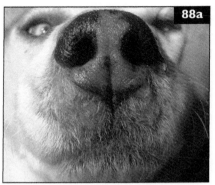
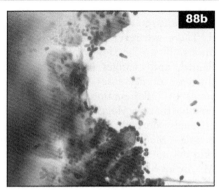

88 A dog presented for nasal depigmentation. Skin lesions are limited to the nose and muzzle (88a). Hair trichograms were negative for *Demodex* mites. Skin cytology revealed these organisms (88b).

i. What are these organisms?

ii. The dog was treated with an appropriate systemic antimicrobial based on the cytologic findings and the nose's pigment returned. What is a possible explanation?

iii. What are other common causes of nasal depigmentation in dogs?

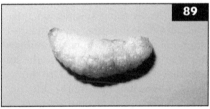

89 This organism (89) was removed from a subcutaneous swelling on the side of the face of a cat.

i. What is the organism?

ii. What is its life cycle, and how did this cat acquire this organism?

iii. When are cats most likely to acquire this infection? This disease has been associated with neurologic signs. How does this occur? What historical finding may be helpful in increasing the index of suspicion of this disease in cats with neurologic signs?

88 i. *Malassezia* spp.

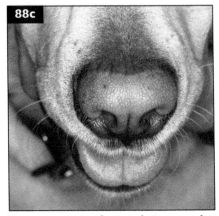

ii. There are several possible explanations. First, the dog's muzzle is inflamed, and changes in pigmentation (increase or decrease) can occur as a result of inflammation. Second, it is possible that the *Malassezia* overgrowth affected normal pigmentation. In people, *Malassezia furfur* causes a skin disease called pityriasis versicolor. *M. furfur* has been found to produce a by-product that blocks tyrosine in melanin production and leads to hypopigmentation in people with this disease. The condition is temporary. This dog's nose regained normal pigment after resolution of the yeast overgrowth.

iii. Trauma, 'snow nose', or seasonal depigmentation (88c), early onset of cutaneous lupus, early onset of cutaneous lymphoma, ketoconazole administration.

89 i. A fly larva of *Cuterebra* spp. (bot flies).

ii. These are obligate parasites of rodents and rabbits. A single female can lay up to thousands of eggs, usually in groups of 10–15 per site. Eggs hatch within a week; this is triggered by a rise in temperature, such as the warm breath of a passing host. Larvae stick to the hair coat and enter the body through mucous membranes. Organisms migrate through tissues using spicules on their surface. Once at the subcutaneous site, they feed on local tissues and after 3–4 weeks create a local swelling with a breathing pore. After undergoing various larval stages they exit the breathing pore, drop to the ground, and burrow into the soil to pupate.

iii. This disease has a seasonal occurrence during late summer to early fall in most geographic locations. Most infestations involve the skin, but larvae can migrate to the eye, trachea, pharynx, and/or upper respiratory tract. Neurologic signs occur when migrating larvae in the respiratory tract gain access to the calvarium via the cribriform plate, middle ear, or other foramen. Previous studies of cats with confirmed CNS *Cuterebra* larvae myiasis were of indoor/outdoor cats presented for depression, lethargy, or seizures during the months of July through September (northern hemisphere). Neurologic examination revealed lateralizing intracranial signs depending on where the larvae traveled. An important historical finding was association with a recent upper respiratory infection, often with severe episodes of sneezing, preceding development of neurologic signs.

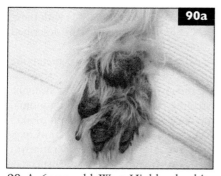

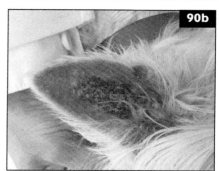

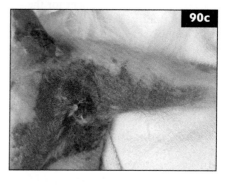

90 A 6-year-old West Highland white terrier dog was presented for the complaint of lethargy, weight loss, and skin lesions. Dermatologic examination revealed lesions on the foot pads (90a), ears (90b), and perineal area (90c). Laboratory evaluation of the dog revealed a normochromic, normocytic, non-regenerative anemia, elevated serum alkaline phosphatase and alanine aminotransferase, and elevated post-prandial bile acid concentrations. ANA testing was negative.

i. What differential diagnoses are ruled out based on the diagnostic testing?
ii. What differential diagnoses should be considered?
iii. Skin biopsy findings revealed the following: diffuse parakeratotic hyperkeratosis, upper level epidermal edema (stratum spinosum and stratum granulosum), vacuolation of keratinocytes, and epidermal hyperplasia. There was a mild superficial perivascular infiltrate in the superficial dermis composed primarily of neutrophils, mast cells, and plasma cells. The pathologist commented that it showed the classic 'red, white, and blue' of 'X' disease. Ultrasound of the liver revealed a small liver with a hyperechoic, reticular pattern surrounding hypoechoic areas ('honeycomb' pattern). What is the most likely diagnosis?

91 Briefly describe the use of interferon (IFN) therapy in veterinary dermatology.

90 i. PF, zinc-responsive skin disease, generic dog food dermatitis. Dogs with these disorders rarely have laboratory abnormalities and/or the clinical signs described for this patient.

ii. SLE, hepatocutaneous syndrome (superficial necrolytic dermatitis, metabolic epidermal necrosis), drug eruption.

iii. Hepatocutaneous syndrome. This is a cutaneous manifestation of a systemic disease. Dogs with liver disease, chronic gastrointestinal disorders, glucagonoma, diabetes mellitus, and pancreatic tumors may develop this unique pattern of skin disease. It has also been reported in dogs on long-term anticonvulsant therapy (e.g. phenobarbital). The pathogenesis is unknown but is related to degeneration of keratinocytes in the upper levels of the epidermis. Nutritional imbalance is suspected. There is no specific treatment for the skin lesions; however, supplementation with high-quality protein (1 egg yolk/4.5 kg), zinc sulfate (10 mg/kg q24h), and fatty acids may be beneficial. Alternatively, infusions of amino acids (500 ml of a 10% solution) IV via a central catheter over 8–10 hours every 7–10 days may be helpful. If there is no response after 4–5 treatments, it is unlikely the patient will improve. If there is resolution of lesions, amino acid therapy is administered as needed. One author (KM) has observed mild resolution of skin lesions in dogs where the underlying metabolic disorder was treated. In most cases, however, the appearance of lesions is associated with severe disease, and most dogs die or are euthanized within 1 year of diagnosis.

91 IFNs are glycoproteins. They are divided into two major groups: type I (IFN-α, IFNω, and IFN-β) and type II (IFN-γ). IFNs are naturally produced and have antiviral, antitumor, and multiple immunomodulatory effects. Recombinant feline IFN omega (rFeIFN-ω) and recombinant canine IFN gamma (CaIFN-γ) have been used for the treatment of dogs with AD; both showed benefit in dogs as an alternative option to immunotherapy. Currently, rCaIFN-γ is licensed for use in Japan for the treatment of AD. rFeIFN-ω has been used to treat a wide range of skin diseases in cats including herpes infection, retrovirus infection, plasma cell pododermatitis, pox virus, feline acne, chronic gingivostomatitis, and pre-operatively and postoperatively in the treatment of feline fibrosarcoma.

92 An 11-year-old female spayed cat with a 5-year history of chronic recurrent bilateral *Malassezia* otitis externa was presented for examination. The most recent episode of otitis had been present for several months and the owner reported the right ear being most affected (odor, copious exudate, presumed pruritus). The cat was presented for examination because of progressive ataxia of 1 months' duration. Neurologic examination revealed decreased sensation on the right side of the face consistent with right facial nerve paralysis. In addition, the ataxia was

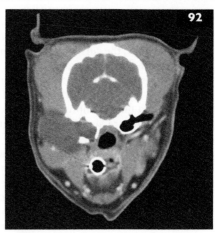

consistent with right-sided vestibular disease. The owner also reported that the cat's purr and meow had changed over the previous month; this was a major concern. Cytologic examination of ear exudate revealed septic inflammation (neutrophils and cocci). The tympanic membrane was not visible on otoscopic examination after cleaning the ear canal. The ear canal appeared to end abruptly.

i. What are the two most likely differential diagnoses? Based on the information provided, which one is most likely?

ii. Imaging of the skull is indicated. The three imaging modalities that could be used in this case are conventional radiographs, CT, and MRI. Briefly discuss key advantages and disadvantages of these three imaging tools.

iii. CT was performed (**92**, post contrast). What are the key findings? Do any explain the change in the cat's vocalizations?

iv. A biopsy of the mass was obtained from soft tissue on the right side of the cat's face. The histologic findings were compatible with an adenocarcinoma. What are the treatment options and prognosis?

93 What organisms comprise the *Staphylococcus intermedius* group (SIG) of bacterial pathogens, and what is the practical significance of this reclassification?

92 i. Vestibular disease due to otitis media and vestibular disease due to neoplasia. Given the history of chronic ear disease, chronic bilateral otitis media is highly suspect; however, the current clinical signs are most likely due to a tumor. Evidence for a tumor includes the age of the cat, acute onset of unilateral worsening, and inability to visualize the tympanic membrane post cleaning with an 'abrupt' ending suggestive of a space-occupying lesion. Changes in the cat's vocalizations are also suggestive of a mass compressing the vocal cords or nerve damage.

ii. CT and MRI are superior to conventional radiography because both provide tomographic images (i.e. slices of the patient). Superimposition of images is avoided using CT and there are enhanced radiographic opacities; conventional radiography only allows for five radiographic opacities. CT allows for larger gray scale and enhancing of contrast between structures. CT allows for visualization of bony structures and radiotherapy treatment planning, if indicated. MRI provides superior soft tissue detail and is the modality of choice for the CNS. One major disadvantage is that there can be geometric distortion of structures, which is problematic for planning radiotherapy treatment.

iii. Large mass extending from the base of the right ear through the right bulla and through the cranium on the right side, creating a mass effect on the caudal pharynx. This most likely explains the changes in the cat's vocalizations. Right otitis media is also noted.

iv. Tumors of the ear tend to be locally invasive and tend not to metastasize. A retrospective review revealed that the most common malignant ear tumors in dogs and cats were ceruminous gland adenocarcinoma, SCC, and carcinoma of undetermined origin. In cats, the prognosis was very poor if neurologic signs were present, if the diagnosis was an SCC or carcinoma, and/or if there was invasion of local tissues.

93 The SIG is comprised of *S. pseudintermedius*, *S. delphini*, and *S. intermedius* based on multilocus sequence analysis. Since the first description in 1976, *S. intermedius* has been considered the primary pathogen of canine pyoderma. In this new classification scheme, the primary pathogen of dogs is *S. pseudintermedius*. From a practical perspective, microbiology laboratories will report culture isolates and sensitivities as 'SIG'. Specific identification of SIG species requires molecular testing and is not performed regularly for clinical isolates. Isolates previously identified as *Staphylococcus intermedius*, but now believed to be *S. pseudintermedius*, are designated in the literature as *[pseud]intermedius*.

94 A 13-year-old male castrated Devon Rex cat presented for rapidly progressive hair loss and increased grooming behavior. The cat was almost completely alopecic on the ventral abdomen, with a 'shiny' appearance to the skin. Waxy, dark debris was noted in the inguinal region and around the claw folds of all four paws (94). Since the cat's last examination 6 months ago, it had lost 1.6 kg. The owner reported that the cat seemed to be eating slightly less and had been more lethargic recently. The cat did not have any previous history of dermatologic abnormalities, it lived indoors, and received year-round flea and tick preventive.

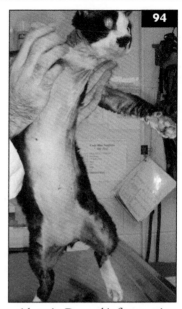

i. Based on the history provided and clinical presentation, what differential diagnoses should be considered? What would be your recommendations for initial diagnostic work-up?

ii. Skin biopsy revealed moderate acanthosis of the epidermis. Dermal inflammation was absent. Most of the hair follicles were in telogen and appeared miniaturized. Abdominal ultrasound revealed a severely mottled pancreas, giving the appearance of an infiltrative process. Given these findings, what is your diagnosis?

iii. With regard to the skin, what is a common secondary complication of this condition?

95 Dog breeds are defined by their conformation and hair coat. The latter has important biological functions and important animal bond functions (i.e. health and emotional benefits from petting the dog). Diseases of the hair follicles impact on both the health of the dog and its appearance.

i. What is a Dermatoscope?

ii. It is commonly believed that puppies 'lose' their puppy coat. It is now known that there are distinct morphologic changes that occur in the hair coat of dogs as they mature. Describe these changes.

iii. What percentage of hair follicles is in telogen in a dog's hair coat?

94 i. The almost complete alopecia and 'shiny' appearance of the skin suggest paraneoplastic alopecia; however, this syndrome can appear very similar to hyperadrenocorticism. The owner should be questioned regarding any history of corticosteroid administration. Skin scraping would be indicated to look for feline demodicosis, a common secondary complication of iatrogenic hyperadrenocorticism. Because of the systemic signs noted (weight loss, lethargy, decreased appetite) additional diagnostics include CBC, serum biochemistry, and urinalysis. Abdominal ultrasound, CT, or MRI is recommended because of the possibility of paraneoplastic alopecia. This condition is reported most commonly with a variety of visceral neoplastic processes, often involving the pancreas. Imaging helps assess whether a solitary tumor or diffuse disease is present.
ii. Paraneoplastic alopecia.
iii. Secondary *Malassezia* overgrowth, reported more so with this condition compared with other internal disease processes. This may contribute to the frequent reports of overgrooming in these animals. In this cat, large numbers of yeast organisms were noted on cytology from the inguinal region and around the claw folds. However, yeast overgrowth is a common finding in Devon Rex cats; it may have been present historically but not deemed problematic as the cat showed no dermatologic abnormalities until the development of paraneoplastic alopecia.

95 i. A portable external microscope that produces high-quality, high-magnification (300X) digital images. It is used for producing live color images of the hair and skin. It is commonly used in human medicine to examine moles.
ii. Hair coat changes were followed in puppies from 10–28 weeks of age using a Dermatoscope and histologic examination of hair follicles via skin biopsy. Three breeds were examined: poodles, Labrador retrievers, Siberian huskies. Results revealed that puppies 'gain an adult hair coat' rather than 'lose their puppy coat'. Over time, the mean number of hair follicles per hair follicle unit increased in all three breeds. In Siberian husky puppies, the growing follicles were predominantly those that produced smaller diameter hair shafts and were curved. This would account for the adult coat, which contains a high number of twisted hair shafts creating a dense undercoat. Labrador retriever puppies had fewer hair follicles per unit than Siberian husky puppies, but the diameter and degree of curvature were similar. As the puppies matured, hairs developed into straight, large diameter hair shafts. This corresponds to the dense coarse hair coat typical of this breed. In poodles, only minimal changes were noted in the diameter and curvature of the hair shafts. In this breed, the changes in the adult hair coat are the result of an increase in the number of hair follicles.
iii. Varies from 50% to >90% depending on the season. One study found that >50% of hair follicles in Labrador retrievers and Siberian husky dogs were in telogen at 28 weeks. In contrast, <10% of poodle dogs had hair follicles in telogen. Observations of >10% of hair follicles in telogen in poodles may suggest a disease state.

96 A 2-year-old male castrated bulldog presented for severe erythema and moderate pruritus of all four paws, the face, and ventrum (96). The owner also reported that patchy alopecia over the dorsum appeared to be progressing to involve more body areas. Clinical signs initially began when the dog was approximately 1 year of age. The only treatment administered had been oral prednisone at a tapering anti-inflammatory dose and oral cephalexin (25 mg/kg q12h for 14 days).

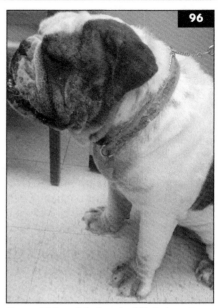

i. What are the possible differential diagnoses for this patient?

ii. Multiple deep skin scrapings identified large numbers of *Demodex canis* mites of all life stages from all four paws, the face, dorsum, and ventrum. How is this form of demodicosis classified?

iii. What are the treatment options for this disease? Note label and off-label options.

97 Compared with dogs, the ear pinnae of cats are consistent in size and shape. Haired skin covers both the convex and concave surfaces and between them is the auricular cartilage, which gives shape to the pinna. This cat (97) was found as a stray and presented for examination for the complaint of 'progressively droopy ears'.

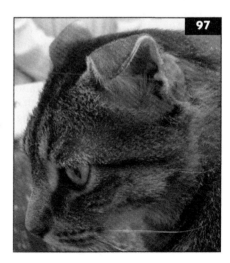

i. What type of cartilage is found in the ear?

ii. What breed of cat has naturally droopy ears?

iii. List common differential diagnoses for damage to ear cartilage of cats.

96 i. Demodicosis, bacterial pyoderma, dermatophytosis, cutaneous adverse reaction to food, AD.
ii. Juvenile-onset generalized demodicosis.
iii. Based on an evidence-based review, several treatment options are deemed efficacious for canine generalized demodicosis. Amitraz dips, currently the only treatment labeled for canine generalized demodicosis, is efficacious at 0.025–0.06% applied once every 7–14 days. In the USA, the product is licensed for use at 0.025% applied once every 14 days. Studies have shown increased efficacy when applied at a higher concentration and/or more frequently. Metaflumizone-amitraz was also labeled for the treatment of canine generalized demodicosis when applied topically once monthly. Additional studies found improved efficacy when the product was applied every 14 days. (**Note:** At the time of publication production of this product has been discontinued in the USA.) Topical moxidectin-imidacloprid has also shown efficacy with weekly application, particularly in patients with more mild disease. Ivermectin has been used effectively since the mid-1980s (0.3–0.6 mg/kg PO q2h). Milbemycin oxime has shown efficacy when administered PO (1–2 mg/kg q24h); however, more rapid and complete response was reported at the higher dosing regimen. Moxidectin (0.2–0.5 mg/kg PO q24h) also demonstrates good efficacy for generalized demodicosis in the dog. Evidence exists to suggest doramectin (0.6 mg/kg SC once every 7 days) as another treatment option.

97 i. Elastic cartilage. This cartilage provides for greater flexibility so that it can withstand greater bending.
ii. Scottish fold. The ear abnormality is the result of a dominant gene mutation that makes the cartilage fold, resulting in pinnae that bend forward.
iii. Trauma, aural hematoma, tumors, hypercortisolemia. Excluding trauma, the most common cause of damage to ear cartilage is an aural hematoma. Acute aural hematomas are easily diagnosed by clinical examination; aspiration of the fluctuant mass will reveal blood, confirming the diagnosis. Untreated and/or recurrent aural hematomas can cause permanent curling fibrosis and deformity of the ear cartilage. 'Droopy ears' are a clinical manifestation of hypercortisolemia caused by naturally occurring adrenal disease or as a result of exogenous corticosteroid administration. It is presumed to be due to weakening of the cartilage and/or collagen. 'Droopy ears' are an increasingly recognized adverse effect of cats receiving potent inhaled glucocorticoids for respiratory disease (e.g. feline asthma).

98 A 3-year-old female spayed German shepherd dog presented for the lesions shown (98). The lesions have been recurrent for 2 years. Skin scrapings and hair trichogram have been negative for *Demodex* mites. Impression smears have revealed cocci and yeast and the lesions respond slowly to concurrent systemic

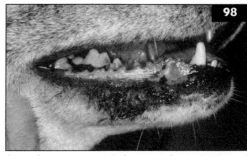

antibiotic and antifungal therapy, but always recur. Culture and sensitivity of the lesions revealed that bacterial resistance was not a complicating factor. Close examination of the lesions reveals odor, pain, erythema, and swelling and crusting of the lips and perioral area. Hairs are trapped in exudate and the lips are depigmented. The dog has a regional lymphadenopathy and a history of dysuria.

i. Describe the clinical distinctions between mucocutaneous pyoderma and bacterial intertrigo (lip fold pyoderma).

ii. What other differential diagnoses need to be considered in this case?

iii. What key histologic criteria would help differentiate the major differential diagnoses?

99 For management of AD, what are the options for humane antipruritic therapy while awaiting a noticeable benefit from immunotherapy (99)?

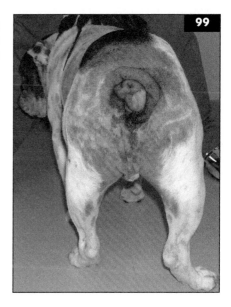

98 i. Mucocutaneous pyoderma and fold pyoderma are clinically very distinctive. The latter is recognized by its location between appositional folds. The folds create a moist, warm environment where bacterial and yeast overgrowth can occur. Lesions rarely extend past the folds. Fold pyoderma is very common. Mucocutaneous pyoderma is less common and does not start in folds nor are the lesions limited to this area. Lesions are symmetrical; the first signs are swelling and erythema followed by crusting, fissuring, and erosions. Lesions often extend to the nasal planum and lips and may involve other mucocutaneous areas such as the prepuce and perineal regions. Facial rubbing can occur and salivary staining is common.
ii. Lupus erythematosus, pemphigus, adverse drug reactions, lymphoma, candidiasis, mucous membrane pemphigoid, cutaneous lymphoma, oral pain (e.g. dental disease).
iii. Key findings: lupus – moderate lichenoid inflammatory infiltrate and basal cell degeneration; pemphgius – subepidermal pustules with acantholysis; mucous membrane pemphigoid – subepidermal clefting; cutaneous lymphoma – tropism of neoplastic lymphocytes for the epidermis and mucous membranes; candidiasis – presence of abundant yeast organisms on special stains; mucocutaneous pyoderma – dermal perivascular to lichenoid infiltrate that does not obscure the basement membrane. Mucocutaneous pyoderma can be difficult to distinguish from lupus as one retrospective study found both to have very similar histologic findings.

99 Bathing to remove allergens, bathing with antimicrobial shampoos to minimize or manage concurrent pruritic microbial overgrowth. Focal application of steroids to intensely pruritic areas (e.g. periocular ophthalmic glucocorticoids, otic glucocorticoids). Essential fatty acid supplements can be helpful, but their action is slow in onset. There is still much controversy about the benefit of antihistamines; as of yet there is inconclusive evidence that they help acute or chronic flares. Essential fatty acids and antihistamines are sometimes used in chronic cases for their steroid-sparing effect. Systemic drugs include cyclosporine (modified), oral prednisone, pentoxifylline, misoprostol, and Chinese herbal extract (steroid sparing). Chinese herbal extracts and other organic compounds may or may not list all of the ingredients. Anecdotally, one of the compounds, liquorice, may have steroid effects; one dog receiving this compound developed calcinosis cutis.

100 A direct mount from a fungal culture colony is shown (100). The culture was from a cat with skin lesions and the colony grew within 7 days of inoculation on to DTM. The gross colony was pale and a red color change developed around it as it was growing.
i. Brief examination of this wet mount reveals two obvious reasons why this is not a pathogen. List them.
ii. Where would the cat have contacted this organism?

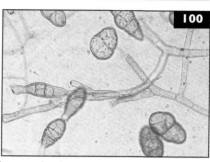

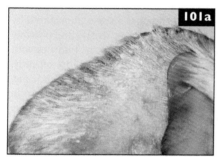

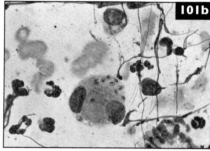

101 A 3-year-old female spayed foxhound-cross dog presents for diffuse, severe crusting dermatosis of several weeks' duration. The owner reports that despite having a ravenous appetite, the dog has also lost weight during the same time period. On physical examination, you note that there is diffuse crusting and silvery-white adherent scaling over the dog's entire body, with thickening of the underlying affected skin and areas of alopecia. Intradermal nodules are also palpated along the pinnae, ears (101a), extremities, and muzzle. Peripheral lymph nodes all palpated enlarged and cranial organomegaly is noted on abdominal palpation. The dog is walking somewhat abnormally; palpation of the limbs identifies swollen and painful joints. There is moderate muscle wasting, most noticeable over the epaxial muscles and hindlimbs.
i. What questions do you have for this owner regarding other pertinent history?
ii. What are your differential diagnoses for this patient?
iii. Cytology from under one of the crusting lesions reveals multiple amastigotes within the cytoplasm of many macrophages (101b). Given this finding, what is your diagnosis? Had cytology failed to identify the disease process, what other diagnostic tests may be considered given the clinical suspicion?
iv. How is this disease managed?

100 i. The hyphae and conidia are pigmented and the conidia have transverse and horizontal septa. This colony is most consistent with an *Alternaria* sp. of fungus. This is commonly confused with macroconidia of *Microsporum canis*.
ii. *Alternaria* spp. are common plant pathogens and are the cause of a wide range of leaf, flower, blossom, and fruit disease. The cat could have contacted this spore inside or outside the house. Also, this spore is commonly found on skin scrapings or surface cytology.

101 i. Travel history, to rule in/out possible infectious diseases. Are any other dogs affected (do they have other pets?). Does the owner have any signs of dermatologic or systemic illness that coincides with the disease development in the dog. Any other history including previous drug administration, history of any dermatologic abnormalities, or signs of illness other than what has been noted recently.
ii. Immune-mediated disease (SLE, PF), epitheliotropic cutaneous lymphoma, dermatophytosis, leishmaniasis, zinc-responsive skin disease, sebaceous adenitis.
iii. Leishmaniasis (*Leishmania infantum*). This is a protozoal disease transmitted by biting sand flies (*Phlebotomus* in Old World, *Lutzomyia* in New World) and possibly other biting insect vectors. It has been reported in the Mediterranean countries with Europe, Africa, South America, and Asia most commonly reported. More recently, the disease has been reported in the USA where it is now considered to be endemic, particularly in foxhound and foxhound-cross dogs. It is an uncommon disease in dogs and rare in cats. When organisms are present on cytology or histopathology and clinical signs are supportive, this finding is diagnostic for the disease. When organisms are not readily present, diagnosis can be confirmed with appropriate serologic evaluation. High titers (e.g. 1/320, 1/640, or 1/1,280) are diagnostic. Cross-reactivity with other infectious diseases has not been reported. If borderline or low titers are noted and there remains clinical suspicion for the disease, lymph node and/or bone marrow aspirates may be helpful for identifying the organisms; amastigotes may still be difficult to find, especially on lymph node aspirate.
iv. The most commonly used treatment protocol is administration of meglumine antimonite (100 mg/kg SC q24h for 4 weeks) along with allopurinol by mouth twice daily for at least 6 months. Treatment efficacy may be monitored via repeated clinical examinations to assess response to treatment as well as repeated qPCR to monitor parasitic load.

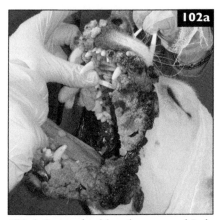 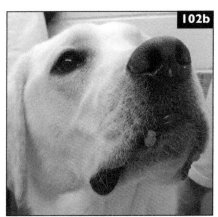

102 A 9-month-old male castrated Labrador retriever dog presented for extensive lesions involving the entire oral cavity (**102a**). Over the last 4 months, a single 'wart'-like lesion had progressed to what is shown. Lesions were present on both the inner and outer labial surfaces bilaterally, along the tongue, hard and soft palates, and extending up the nasal philtrum. The masses did not affect the dog's ability to eat or play; however, lesions were easily traumatized. The owner's complaint at the time of the visit was "my home looks like a crime scene" due to the amount of bleeding that occurred whenever the lesions were traumatized or the dog shook its head. In addition, the owner reported a foul odor from the dog's mouth.

i. What is your clinical diagnosis?

ii. What immediate concerns do you have regarding this dog's overall health?

iii. What are possible treatment options? This is the dog after treatment (**102b**).

103 What is silver sulfadiazine (AgSD)?

102 i. Severe oral papillomatosis (rare).

ii. Although the exact mechanism resulting in either spontaneous regression or spread of papillomas is not known, spontaneous regression is suspected to be associated with the presence of CD4$^+$ and CD8$^+$ lymphocytes. In this case, regression had not occurred after several months, raising serious concerns about a defect in the dog's immune response. Humoral immunity may also be affected; severe papillomatosis has been reported in beagles with IgA deficiency.

iii. In this case, surgical debulking is needed: cold steel, cryosurgery, or electrosurgery using a carbon dioxide laser. Recombinant canine oral papillomavirus vaccination has been beneficial for disease prophylaxis as well as for treatment of oral papillomatosis in dogs; however, caution is warranted as cutaneous neoplasms may form at the injection site, albeit years later. One study reported on the efficacy of azithromycin therapy for regression of canine oral papillomatosis; a dose of 10 mg/kg daily led to a decrease in clinical scores of the papillomas. Other treatment options include systemic chemotherapy with single-agent vincristine, cyclophosphamide, or doxorubicin. Administration of interferon has been investigated; however, at low oral doses treatment has not been highly effective. In people, the use of immunostimulants such as imiquimod has been beneficial; the medication causes cytokine induction and stimulation of the humoral and cell-mediated immune systems that leads to papilloma regression. Cimetidine, which also acts as an immunostimulant, has had some success as an adjunct treatment for various papillomavirus conditions in people. Anecdotally, topical imiquimod 5% cream (applied q24–48h until lesions regress) has been beneficial in dogs. Also, cimetidine (20–30 mg/kg q12h) has been efficacious in many cases of papillomatosis in dogs. This dog responded to a combination of surgical debulking, imiquimod cream for several months, and cimetidine. Ultimately, the lesions recurred and the owner elected euthanasia as permanent remission could not be induced.

103 A combination of silver and sulfadiazine. It is a water soluble cream that has broad-spectrum antibacterial activity. AgSD serves as a reservoir of silver in the wound and slowly releases silver ions. The proposed mechanism of action is that AgSD binds to cell DNA, resulting in membrane damage. The binding of AgSD to the base pairs in the bacterial DNA helix inhibits transcription, leading to inhibition of bacterial growth. Currently, AgSD is used widely as a cream or as compounded drops to treat a wide range of infections in veterinary dermatology, especially multidrug-resistant *Pseudomonas* ear infections. The use of silver in nanotechnology is being explored, as nanotechnology can change the chemical, physical, and optical properties of silver and offer new biomedical options.

104 A Wood's lamp is a common diagnostic tool in small animal dermatology.
i. When was the lamp invented, and when was it first used?
ii. What are the physics behind the use of the Wood's lamp?
iii. What is the most common use of this tool in veterinary dermatology?

105 A 3-year-old female spayed goldendoodle dog presented for severe hindlimb swelling (**105**), progressive cutaneous bruising, and fever. The dog also had a recent history of gastrointestinal upset (including hematochezia and hematemesis) following an episode of dietary indiscretion approximately 1 week prior to the development of skin lesions. She had been treated by her primary care veterinarian with various anti-emetics and metronidazole. On physical examination, the dog was diffusely erythematous and severely pruritic; several areas of self-trauma were noted, particularly along the cervical region. Multiple areas of diffuse ecchymotic hemorrhage were identified; diascopy was performed, which did not identify blanching of the skin. CBC revealed peripheral eosinophilia. The only abnormality noted on serum biochemistries was moderate hypoalbuminemia.

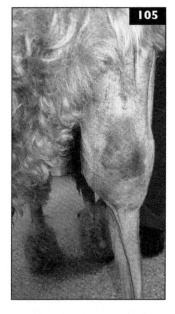

i. What other diagnostics would you consider performing for this patient?
ii. A skin biopsy of this patient showed severe superficial and deep, perivascular to diffuse eosinophilic dermatitis. Several degranulating eosinophils were noted around collagen fibers forming 'flame figures'. Dermal edema was noted to be moderate and many vessels were markedly dilated. What is the diagnosis based on the biopsy and clinical findings?
iii. What is this condition, and what has been reported about it in dogs?

104 i. 1903 by Robert W Wood. The first description of its use for diagnosis of fungal infections was in 1925.

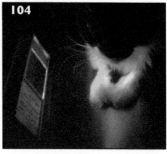

ii. It emits long-wave radiation generated from a high-pressure mercury arc. The lamp contains a compound filter made of barium silicate with 9% nickel oxide (called the Wood's filter), which blocks all light rays except for those between 320 and 400 nm with a peak at 354 nm.

iii. As a screening tool for detection of *Micro-sporum canis* infections (**104**). Other dermatophyte species that fluoresce a bright green color include *M. distorum* and *M. audouinni*. *Trichophyton schoeleinni* organisms fluoresce a dull blue and some variants of *M. gypsum* will fluoresce a dull yellow. *M. canis* is the predominant veterinary pathogen that fluoresces. The compound that causes fluorescence in *Microsporum* species is a pteridine.

105 i. Clotting times (prothrombin time and partial prothrombin time, buccal mucosal bleeding time), skin biopsy if there are no contraindications, FNA of affected area.

ii. Eosinophilic dermatitis (eosinophilic cellulitis, Wells-like syndrome).

iii. Wells syndrome is another term for eosinophilic cellulitis in people. In dogs, the disease process is considered to be rare; it is suspected to be due to a severe hypersensitivity reaction, as seasonality has been noted in several reported cases. A retrospective study identified three different groups of dogs with similar histologic features on skin biopsy. The first group was composed of dogs previously treated for gastrointestinal illness prior to the development of skin lesions. The second group had concurrent gastrointestinal illness at the time of cutaneous lesion development. The third group had solely cutaneous lesions in the absence of gastrointestinal illness. Between groups one and two, previous exposure to various medications, gastrointestinal upset (vomiting and/or diarrhea, often with hematemesis and/or hematochezia), and hypoalbuminemia were common findings. Possible drug reaction or association is suspected to be a potential cause of disease development. Dogs can recover from the condition if treatment is initiated as soon as possible; typically, high anti-inflammatory to low immunosuppressive doses of corticosteroids is beneficial plus supportive care for any concurrent gastrointestinal illness. Monitoring for sepsis and dehydration is imperative.

106 A 1.5-year-old cat was presented for acute intense pruritus of the caudal dorsum and medial aspect of the hindlimbs (106). Physical examination revealed multifocal areas of patchy alopecia on the dorsal lumbosacral region and complete hair loss on the entire caudal ventrum and inguinal areas. The cat was very sensitive to touch anywhere around its hindquarters. The

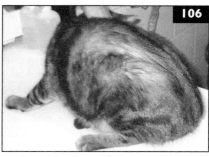

owner reported that the cat had no access to other animals and lived on the seventh floor of an apartment building but did occasionally sit on the outdoor patio. The owner moved into this apartment 5 months ago and the pruritus began within 4–6 weeks of the move. Skin scraping was negative for mites and flea combing did not reveal any live fleas or flea feces.

i. Based on the physical examination findings, what condition do you initially choose to treat?
ii. How can you explain your treatment plan to the owner?

107 A 3-year-old male neutered mixed-breed dog presents with non-pruritic bilateral symmetrical alopecia along the trunk and proximal extremities of 4 months' duration. Clinical examination shows the blue hairs to be affected (107). Alopecia is predominantly restricted to the dorsolateral trunk and proximal extremities. Other cutaneous findings include comedones and dry, non-

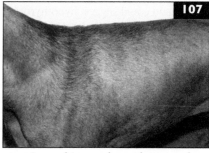

adherent scales in areas of hair loss. Skin scrapings, skin cytology, dermatophyte culture, CBC, and serum chemistries are all negative or within laboratory reported normal ranges.

i. Are there any additional questions you would like answered?
ii. What is the most likely diagnosis, and how does it develop?
iii. What diagnostic test(s) would confirm your clinical suspicion?

106 i. Flea allergy dermatitis/hypersensitivity.

ii. Some owners find it hard to believe that fleas are the underlying cause when no fleas are found on physical examination. Knowledge of the flea life cycle may help. A host is required for food and protection; fleas spend their entire adult life on their host. Eggs are laid on the animal and fall into the environment where they go through three larval and one pupal stage. Fleas can remain in the pupal stage for over 100 days. If the owner's apartment had previously housed animals who were infested with fleas, the cat may have provided the right stimuli (temperature, vibration, carbon dioxide) to cause emergence of the adult fleas, leading to infestation.

Flea-allergic animals often develop highly effective grooming skills to remove parasites that are causing them intense discomfort. This helps explain why a flea-allergic animal will often have no fleas. The reaction of the cat to touch on the hindquarters further demonstrates the extreme sensitivity that fleas can cause. One study found that approximately 40% of cats responded to flea control measures alone even when obvious evidence of fleas was absent. Flea control medications are generally safe and well tolerated, making the downsides to treatment very few. Response to judicious application of monthly flea control medication for at least 3 months in combination with environmental control will help to confirm the diagnosis.

107 i. Is the dog polyuric, polydipsic, polyphagic? Constantly panting? Gained weight? When was the dog neutered? Are other animals in the household similarly affected? Any littermates similarly affected? Affirmative answers to questions 1–3 might suggest hyperadrenocorticism (atypical age of onset for endogenous disease). Weight gain could suggest hypothyroidism. Castration-responsive dermatosis is rare but plausible. Although dermatophyte culture was 'negative', similarly affected pets would raise suspicion of a false-negative test result. Familial history of a similar problem among littermates or parents would suggest an inherited skin disease.

ii. CDA, a genetic alopecic condition of 'dilute' (blue or fawn) coat colors. Affected dogs are born with a normal coat, but thinning and alopecia progress as they mature. Alopecia begins with color dilute hairs along the dorsal back and progresses down the lateral trunk. Secondary bacterial folliculitis, generalized scaling, comedone formation, and hyperpigmentation are common sequelae. Regrown hairs are usually deformed. A genetic defect (D locus of color dilute gene) causing follicular and melanin dysplasia results in dysplastic hair shafts. Although most common in Doberman pinscher dogs, any breed can be affected.

iii. A trichogram shows melanin clumping and distortion of hair shaft anatomy. Aggregated macromelanosomes in the basal cell layer of the epidermis and follicular epithelium, hair matrix cells, hair shaft, and sebaceous glands, with varying degrees of follicular dysplasia and cystic follicles, may be seen on skin biopsy.

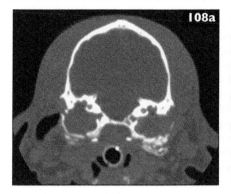

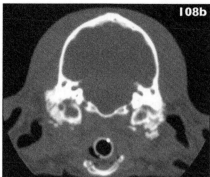

108 An 8-year-old female spayed cocker spaniel dog is presented for a 3-year history of bilateral otitis externa. Physical examination reveals a mild waxy discharge bilaterally. There is resistance to opening the dog's mouth for oral examination, which appears largely normal. Otic examination is

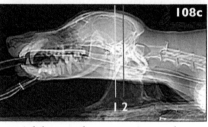

normal other than the presence of a white material deep to the tympanic membrane, which appears intact. CT of the skull is performed (108a–c).

i. What are the imaging findings?

ii. What are the differential diagnoses and associated pathophysiology?

iii. What are the recommendations for intervention, possible complications, and the prognosis?

109 A 4-year-old male castrated Scottish terrier dog presents for the patch of alopecia shown (107). The owners do not report pruritus, monthly spot-on topical flea control is used year round, and the dog does not have any other dermatologic abnormalities. Based on the appearance of the lesion, what questions should be asked of the owners?

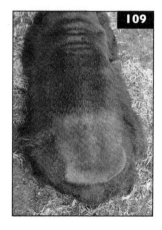

108 i. Both tympanic bullae are expanded with thin and partially disrupted bony margins. There is extensive new bone proliferation, most prominent medial and ventral to the bulla and along the retroarticular process to the temporal bone. Both bullae are filled with enhancing soft tissue material.

ii. Bilateral aural cholesteatoma, bilateral severe chronic otitis media, or neoplasia. Aural cholesteatomas are epidermoid cysts forming within the middle ear. They are composed of keratin debris surrounded by keratinizing stratified squamous epithelium. These can be congenital or acquired; they are most often reported as a complication of chronic otitis media/externa in dogs. Once the cyst is formed it can expand with accumulation of keratin debris and/or sebaceous material, resulting in various degrees of inflammatory response.

iii. Curative-intent treatment involves surgical excision of the cholesteatoma. Surgical approach is based on extent of disease, but often total ear canal ablation and lateral bulla osteotomy and/or ventral bulla osteotomy are considered. Complications include facial nerve injury, excessive hemorrhage, abscess, and seroma formation. Recurrence after surgery is reported in 50% of dogs. Risk factors for recurrence include inability to open the mouth or neurologic signs on admission, and temporal bone lysis on CT. Median survival time of dogs with neurologic signs or inability to open the mouth is 16 months. Encroachment of the temporomandibular joint as documented on the CT scans in this patient likely accounts for the difficulty opening her mouth, and contributes to the guarded prognosis.

109 The region of alopecia is very well demarcated. An important question to ask is when they last remembered the dog to have hair in this area and whether or not the hair coat has been clipped since. This pattern is common in post-clipping alopecia. Other differentials include endocrine alopecia, superficial bacterial pyoderma, demodicosis, and dermatophytosis, but the well-demarcated nature of the alopecic region makes these highly unlikely. This dog had a surgical repair of a cranial cruciate ligament rupture 2 years prior to presentation. At the time of surgery, an epidural had been administered for pain control. While the area clipped for surgery regrew hair normally, the epidural site remained alopecic. This is a cosmetic condition, which may be permanent or transient in nature; it can take upwards of 18 months or longer for some dogs to completely regrow their hair coat. No treatment is required.

110 An 8-year-old female spayed mixed-breed dog presented for recurrent bacterial pyoderma of several months' duration. The owner also noted that the dog appeared to be gaining weight recently and was slightly lethargic. On closer examination, these lesions were noted multifocally along the abdomen and trunk (110a). Routine CBC showed thrombocytosis and lymphopenia. Serum biochemistries showed severely elevated alkaline phosphatase and mild

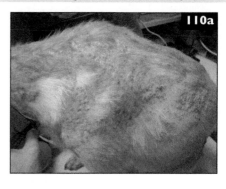

elevations in alanine aminotransferase and cholesterol. The dog had no history of any previous medical abnormalities, including dermatologic problems.

i. What is the most likely diagnosis for this patient?

ii. What cutaneous manifestations are associated with this disease process?

111 A 7-year-old male castrated Labrador retriever dog presented for a solitary hyperpigmented mass on the cranial thoracic region of the dorsum (111). The dermal mass was approximately 2 cm in diameter, hyperpigmented, well circumscribed, and somewhat soft on palpation. No other clinical signs were reported by the owners and no other lesions were found on physical examination of the dog.

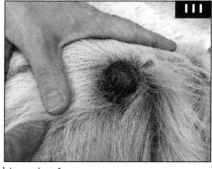

i. What are the differential diagnoses for this patient?

ii. On FNA of the mass, a moderate amount of local hemorrhage was noted. Within a few minutes, the dog developed urticaria, edema, and erythema surrounding the mass. Given this additional history, what is the most likely diagnosis for the mass?

iii. Which breeds are predisposed to this type of cutaneous mass?

110 i. Hyperadrenocorticism. Because the dog had no previous history of glucocorticoid administration, spontaneous hyperadrenocorticism is most likely. Pituitary-dependent hyperadrenocorticism accounts for approximately 85% of canine hyperadrenocorticism cases (pituitary microadenomas) and 15% are due to a functional adrenal tumor. Other possible causes include ectopic ACTH secretion or

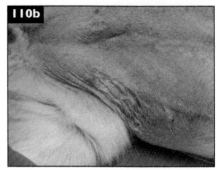

ectopic/hyperactive eutopic adrenocortical receptors, but these are extremely rare occurrences in dogs.

ii. Alopecia, typically bilaterally symmetrical and sparing the head and extremities. Failure to regrow hair following shaving or grooming is also reported. Alopecia is due to steroid-induced atrophy of the hair follicle and pilosebaceous unit. Comedone formation may be noted, particularly around the mammae and dorsal and ventral midlines. Keratin plugged follicles occur due to accumulation of debris in an atrophic follicle, or may be secondary to demodicosis or bacterial pyoderma. Recurrent bacterial pyoderma in a dog with no prior history may be the only presenting sign when 'classic' clinical signs (i.e. polyuria/polydipsia) are absent. Skin infections may be further complicated by seborrhea. Unless there are secondary pruritic triggers (e.g. pyoderma, *Malassezia* overgrowth) pruritus is uncommon; inflammation is masked by excess circulating corticosteroids. Other dermatologic abnormalities include thin, atonic skin (**110b**), calcinosis cutis and milia, hyperpigmentation, phlebectasia, and bruising.

111 i. Neoplasia (basal cell carcinoma, hair follicle tumor, apocrine gland tumor, hemangioma, hemangiosarcoma, MCT, cutaneous lymphoma, plasmacytoma, melanoma); non-neoplastic mass including local hemorrhage, foreign body reaction, or, less likely, infectious etiologies.

ii. MCT. The adverse reaction exhibited by the dog following aspiration is known as Darier's sign.

iii. Australian cattle dog, beagle, Boston terrier, boxer, bullmastiff, bull terrier, cocker spaniel, dachshund, English bulldog, fox terrier, golden retriever, Labrador retriever, pug, Rhodesian ridgeback, schnauzer, shar-pei, Staffordshire terrier, Weimaraner. In these breeds, the disease usually presents as a solitary cutaneous mass; however, the following dog breeds most frequently present with multiple tumors: boxer, golden retriever, pug, shar-pei, and Weimaraner.

112 i. How is hyperadrenocorticism definitively diagnosed in the dog?
ii. What treatment options are available for consideration?

113 An owner whose hobby is sled dog racing presented one of 10 dogs for examination. The owner reported that all dogs were showing similar clinical signs and this dog was representative of the entire group (**113a**). The dogs showed moderate to severe pruritus and self-trauma of 1 year's duration. There were no cats on the premises. The owner reported that she was also pruritic. The dogs live with the owner and have full access to her home through a dog door. The dog door leads to an outdoor pen that contains doghouses. The owner uses straw for bedding and changes it weekly. All dogs receive monthly spot-on flea control. Skin scrapings were negative for *Demodex* mites. Cytology of the excoriated areas revealed overgrowth of *Malassezia* and neutrophils with intracellular cocci. Flea combing did not identify any fleas; however, this organism (**113b**) was found under a mat of hair.

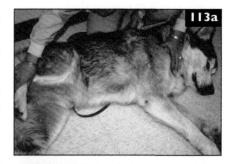

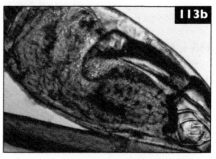

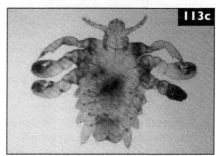

i. What is this organism?
ii. What is the organism in **113c**?
iii. What is the most likely cause of the dog's pruritus? What are the treatment options?

112 i. Screening tests include urine cortisol–creatinine ratio, ACTH stimulation test, and low-dose dexamethasone suppression test. Low-dose dexamethasone suppression tests can determine 'is this hyperadrenocorticism' and 'what is the etiology'. Lack of suppression for the entire 8-hour test period is compatible with hyperadrenocorticism; in 60–65% of dogs with pituitary-dependent hyperadrenocorticism, the 4-hour plasma cortisol concentration will suppress, but then 'escape' by 8 hours. Suppression should not occur in dogs with functional adrenal tumors. If suppression does not occur at either time point, a high-dose dexamethasone suppression test may be performed to differentiate. Desmopressin stimulation has been described as a potentially useful differentiating test. More commonly, advanced imaging techniques (abdominal ultrasound, CT, MRI) are utilized to evaluate the adrenal glands. CT or MRI may be used to evaluate the pituitary gland, particularly when neurologic abnormalities are reported.

ii. Trilostane and mitotane administration are medical options for dogs with PDH. Ketoconazole decreases steroidogenesis by inhibiting the cytochrome p-450 enzyme system; it has been effective in some dogs. Selegiline, bromocriptine, and cyproheptadine have all been evaluated as treatment options, but are not effective. Adrenalectomy is the treatment of choice for adrenal tumors as it may offer the potential for cure. Other options include pituitary radiation therapy and hypophysectomy; these options may be considered in patients with neurologic abnormalities.

113 i. Louse nit. The major differential for this organism is a *Cheyletiella* egg; however, these are not tightly glued to the hairs and are smaller.

ii. A human louse, *Phthirus pubis*. This would explain the owner's pruritus but not the dog's, since lice are species specific.

iii. Combined bacterial and yeast infections are likely contributing to the dog's pruritus; however, the underlying trigger is louse infestation. Dogs can be infested by two lice species: sucking louse (*Linognathus setosus*) and biting louse (*Trichodectes canis*). Louse infestations are most common in situations of overcrowding and poor hygiene. In this case, the bedding should be changed more frequently to minimize mechanical transmission. Lice spend their entire life cycle on the host and only live for 1–2 days off the host; attention to possible objects that could allow for fomite transmission (straw bedding, rugs, blankets) is necessary. Treat all in-contact animals. Louse nits need to be removed from the hair coat or else reinfestation can occur. Clipping the hair coat of long-haired animals is effective, as is aggressive bathing to loosen nits. Anecdotally, vinegar and water rinses 1:1 have been used to soften the cement attachment to the hairs. Aggressively bathe dogs to remove nits and apply a whole body insecticide rinse. Spot-on products (e.g. fipronil, selamectin, imidacloprid) have been used successfully to treat individual animal infestations, but are not recommended for multi-animal outbreaks or in animals with dense hair coats.

114 What is the difference between acanthosis, acantholysis, and acantholytic cell?

115 Immunohistochemical markers are used to aid the pathologist in identifying the specific cell type involved in a disease process. Specific cell types possess patterns of immunohistochemical staining (typically reported as positive or negative), which identify the various cell types involved. This process is used most frequently for neoplastic processes to determine the cell or tissue of origin (from personal communication, Texas A&M University College of Veterinary Medicine and Biomedical Sciences Pathology Department). Match the following immunohistochemical cell markers with the cell type identified:

i:	c-kit	A:	all leukocytes
ii:	CD1	B:	striated muscle, smooth muscle
iii:	CD3	C:	neurons, neuroendocrine cells including Schwann and Merkel's cells
iv:	CD11b/d	D:	epithelium
v:	CD11a/CD18	E:	dendritic cells
vi:	CD20/CD79a	F:	basement membrane
vii:	CD45	G:	mesenchymal cells including fibroblasts, endothelial cells, myoepithelial cells, smooth and skeletal muscle, melanocytes, and various inflammatory cells
viii:	collagen IV	H:	macrophages
ix:	cytokeratin	I:	leukocytes except erythroid cells and plasma cells
x:	desmin	J:	mast cells
xi:	melan A	K:	skeletal muscle
xii:	myoglobulin	L:	T cells
xiii:	neuron-specific enolase	M:	melanocytes
xiv:	synaptophysin	N:	neuroendocrine cells
xv:	vimentin	O:	B cells

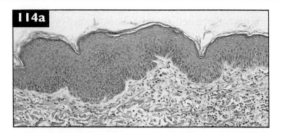

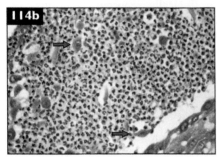

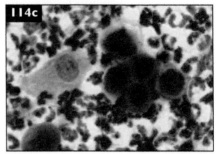

114 Acanthosis refers to an increase in the thickness of the stratum spinosum of the epidermis (**114a**). It is a common finding in inflammatory skin diseases. Acantholysis refers to disruption and separation of the keratinocytes (arrows) of the epidermis in the stratum spinosum. It is caused by lysis of the intercellular cement. It is most commonly observed in pustular diseases, particularly severe bacterial pyoderma and PF, where it is a hallmark feature of the disease (**114b**). Acantholytic cell refers to the individual separated cells that result from the process of acantholysis. In severe bacterial pyoderma, cells tend to be seen singly or in small groups. In PF, these cells are commonly observed in rafts or groups. The dark blue cells shown (**114c**) are an example of a raft of cells. These cells can be readily observed on skin cytology from a pustule in a patient with PF.

115 i. = J; ii. = E; iii. = L; iv. = H; v. = A; vi. = O; vii. = I; viii. = F; ix. = D; x. = B; xi. = M; xii. = K; xiii. = C; xiv. = N; xv. = G.

116 A 6-year-old male castrated DLH cat presents for management of a chronic allergic skin disease. The cat is morbidly obese, weighing 10.45 kg (23 pounds) and with a body condition score of 9/9. The cat has previously been managed with injectable long-acting corticosteroid administration due to the owner's inability to administer pills to

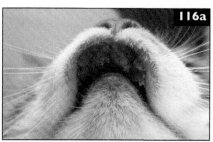

the animal. Recently, the cat has become diabetic and requires insulin in addition to dietary management for diabetes mellitus (DM). On physical examination, the cat has a large indolent ulcer involving the upper lip bilaterally (116a) as well as multiple eosinophilic plaques along the ventral abdomen. The cat is moderately pruritic and has developed self-induced alopecia along the most caudal portion of the ventral abdomen (the only portion of the abdomen the cat can reach).

i. What are the options for controlling the immediate pruritus in this animal?

ii. With regard to long-term management of the allergic skin disease, what options may be considered and what difficulties do you face diagnostically with this patient?

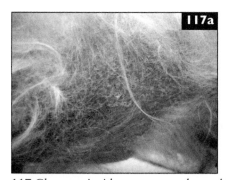 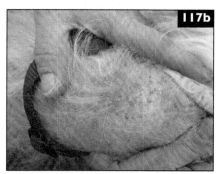

117 Glucocorticoids are commonly used in veterinary dermatology.

i. What are the common side-effects of long-term topical glucocorticoid use (117a, b)?

ii. What are the common side-effects of systemic glucocorticoid use?

116 i. Corticosteroid administration is not a viable option given the history and development of DM; insulin resistance is a potential complication. Antibiotic administration may be beneficial; many of these lesions respond well to antibiotic administration alone. If antibiotic administration does not alleviate the cat's pruritus, additional therapy with cyclosporine is the next best option. Although DM is a reported cyclosporine side-effect, it does appear to be less diabetogenic compared with corticosteroids.

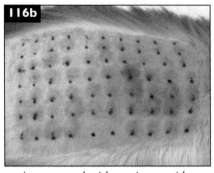

ii. Skin scraping and cytology should be performed to rule out generalized demodicosis and secondary infections, respectively, as complicating factors. Assuming the cat is receiving year-round adulticide flea prevention, a diet trial would also be indicated; however, this may be difficult with concurrent DM. Therefore, treatment should be aimed at managing presumed AD. This could include administration of fatty acids and antihistamines (adjunct or sole therapy) and cyclosporine or pursuing allergy testing and ASIT. (Note complications with cyclosporine above.) If the cat's appetite decreases with cyclosporine administration (fairly common albeit transient adverse effect), development of hepatic lipidosis would be a concern. ASIT would be the safest option long term. A weight loss plan should be recommended for the cat; DM may be transient due to the previous steroid administration. In this cat, ASIT was pursued based on the IDT shown here (**116b**).

117 i. Scaling of the skin, thinning of the skin, focal alopecia, focal hyper-pigmentation, easily bruised skin, easily torn skin, telangiectasia, follicular inclusion cysts, comedones, calcinosis cutis or milia formation, focal drug reaction to the commercial product or base, depigmentation of skin, elevations of serum chemistry parameters, blunting of ACTH stimulation test.

ii. Polyuria, polydipsia, polyphagia, weight gain, panting, muscle weakness, muscle wasting, joint laxity/injury, inappropriate urination, depression, behavior changes, iatrogenic hyperadrenocorticism, cystitis, 'silent' urinary tract infections, gastric ulceration, vomiting, diarrhea, liver and metabolic changes (e.g. diabetes mellitus), hair loss, calcinosis cutis, scaling of the skin, skin infections (bacterial, dermatophytosis), demodicosis, comedones. Less commonly, steroid-related aggression and mood changes can occur in dogs.

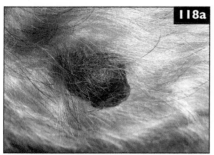 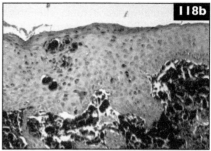

118 This lesion (118a) was found on the dorsum of a 3-year-old dog during an annual examination. The owner was unaware of the lesion. It was removed via excisional biopsy and a photomicrograph of the skin biopsy is shown (118b).
i. What are the diagnosis and prognosis?
ii. How does the site affect the prognosis?
iii. What is the most recent non-interventional therapy?

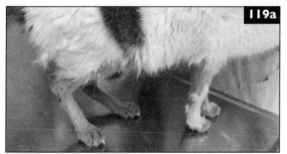 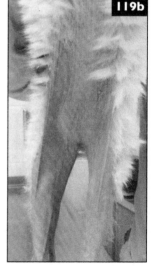

119 A 14-year-old male castrated cat presented for lethargy, decreased appetite, and weight loss of 3 months' duration. The owner also noted that the cat was losing a large amount of hair, particularly along the ventrum and limbs (119a). Large sheets of exfoliated scale were present throughout the skin, particularly in areas of near complete alopecia (119b).
i. What diagnostic tests are indicated, and why?
ii. What are your differential diagnoses based on the clinical appearance?
iii. What neoplastic processes have been implicated in association with this clinical appearance?

118 i. Dermal melanocytoma, the most common melanocytic tumor of dogs. They are usually solitary, circumscribed, brown to black, and alopecic. The size varies from 0.5–4.0 cm. The prognosis is good if wide surgical margins are obtained.

ii. Canine melanocytic lesions can occur anywhere on the body. They occur more commonly in darkly pigmented dogs. Clinically, it can be difficult to differentiate between a benign and a malignant melanoma; however, location of the lesion may be important. The vast majority of oral melanomas and approximately two-thirds of melanomas from the digits are malignant. In contrast, most melanomas from the skin are benign. Recently, a malignant melanoma from the perianal region of the dog was reported; this is a very unusual location for a melanoma.

iii. The licensure of a DNA vaccine for dogs with oral melanoma in 2010. The vaccine contains a DNA plasmid containing a gene for human tyrosinase, a protein found on both human and canine melanoma cancer cells. In a study involving 58 dogs with stage II or stage III oral melanoma, dogs receiving the vaccine post surgical debulking had a significantly longer survival time than did control dogs. Side-effects included minimal to mild pain at the site of injection, and a single dog developed vitiligo.

119 i. CBC, serum biochemistry, and urinalysis to determine whether obvious metabolic abnormalities exist. Ultrasound, CT, or MRI of the abdomen for structural abnormalities or masses. Skin biopsy to determine if clinical findings are due to a primary dermatologic problem or if skin changes are associated with cutaneous manifestation of a systemic disease.

ii. Paraneoplastic alopecia, superficial necrolytic dermatitis (although typically, less alopecia is present), hyperadrenocorticism, feline thymoma-associated exfoliative dermatitis, dermatophytosis, PF, cutaneous epitheliotropic T-cell lymphoma, SLE, EM, demodicosis.

iii. The most likely diagnosis is paraneoplastic alopecia. The 'shiny' appearance of the skin (associated with complete alopecia in the absence of inflammation) with large amounts of scale is visually distinctive. The pattern of hair loss is also supportive of the disease. This type of paraneoplastic syndrome may be associated with any underlying visceral neoplasia; however, pancreatic cancer is most frequently reported. Hepatocellular carcinoma has also been associated with feline paraneoplastic alopecia. The combination of alopecia on the face and moderate exfoliative dermatitis is supportive of feline thymoma-associated exfoliative dermatitis and cutaneous epithelial T-cell lymphoma. These conditions typically have a more diffuse pattern of scaling and alopecia compared with cats with paraneoplastic alopecia; the distribution of alopecia is typically ventral. The prognosis for cases of feline paraneoplastic alopecia is poor.

120 A 3-year-old female spayed mixed-breed dog presented for multiple erythematous, nodular skin lesions affecting the haired skin of the muzzle, flanks, and ventral abdomen as well as several mucocutaneous junctions (eye lids, vulva, lips) (120a). The nodules were minimally pruritic, raised with an umbilicated center, and primarily non-ulcerated at the time of presentation.

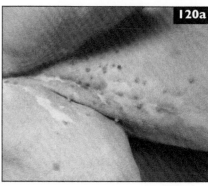

i. What are the differential diagnoses for this patient?

ii. Skin biopsy of the lesions revealed 'focally extensive areas of severe infiltration of neutrophils and macrophages with fewer eosinophils and lymphocytes in the dermis. The infiltration extends from the superficial to deep dermis and focally into the subcutaneous adipose tissue. In several sections within the nodular aggregation of pyogranulomatous inflammation, there are few extracellular and intrahistiocytic, round to crescent-shaped, non-staining 5–20 µm diameter yeast with occasional narrow-based budding. Yeasts are surrounded by a clear, 5–10 µm wide capsule giving the organisms a 'soap bubble' appearance. The organisms are noted to be refractile.' What is the diagnosis for this patient?

iii. How does this organism differ with regard to canine and feline infection?

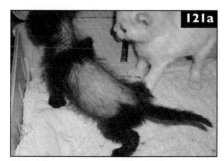 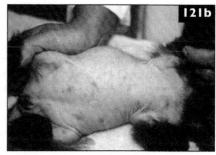

121 These two 6-week-old kittens are littermates (121a). The abdomen of the black kitten, approximately 1 month later, is shown (121b). What is the diagnosis?

120 i. Infectious: deep fungal including blastomycosis, cryptococcosis, histoplasmosis, coccidioidomycosis; atypical bacterial including botryomycosis, mycobacterial infection, nocardiosis, actinomycosis, canine leproid granuloma; inflammatory: cutaneous histiocytosis, sterile pyogranuloma/granuloma syndrome; neoplasia: cutaneous epitheliotropic T-cell lymphoma.

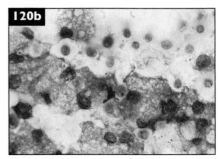

ii. Cryptococcosis (**120b** shows organisms from an impression smear).

iii. Disease is acquired from the environment via inhalation of infective spores or yeast organisms. It is not considered to be contagious or zoonotic. In dogs, it occurs in individuals typically <4 years old. Major organs involved are the nasal cavity, CNS, and eyes. CNS signs include meningitis, meningoencephalitis, head tilt, nystagmus, paresis, ataxia, circling, and seizures. Ocular changes include optic neuritis, retinal hemorrhage, blindness, anterior uveitis, and periorbital swelling. The nasal cavity can be involved but respiratory signs are often subclinical or very mild; rhinosinusitis is not typically reported in the dog. Cutaneous lesions are considered to be a marker of disseminated disease. Cryptococcosis is more common in young cats. Common signs include sneezing, mucopurulent nasal discharge, mandibular lymphadenopathy, and possibly otitis media. CNS signs are variable and include depression, changes in behavior and temperament, seizures, circling, vestibular signs, and blindness. Ocular changes are a sentinel sign of CNS involvement. Compared with dogs, where cutaneous signs are less common, cats often present with papules and nodules, particularly involving the nasal planum.

121 Congenital hypotrichosis. This condition is due to a lack of adnexa in the regions where they are normally found. It is a rare condition, which is noted at birth or shortly thereafter. It is believed to be caused by a spontaneous genetic mutation. This mutation has been reported in kittens before, but with concurrent congenital oligodontia of both the deciduous and permanent teeth. It has also been reported in a litter of Birman kittens that had concurrent thymic aplasia. This kitten had normal deciduous and permanent teeth. Long-term management required additional moisturizing of the skin by the owners and careful restriction of the kitten from excessively sunny areas to prevent solar-induced actinic damage.

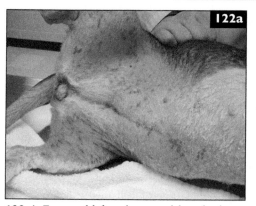
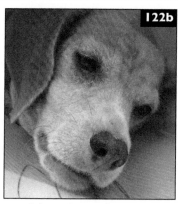

122 A 7-year-old female spayed beagle dog presented for a 3-month progressive history of severe pruritus and excessive scaling. The dog was pruritic to the point that massive self-trauma was present in the form of linear excoriation and erosions (**122a**). The owner had noted that the dog's nose was beginning to turn pink compared with its normal black appearance (**122b**). Previous treatment for ectoparasites and infections had not been beneficial.

i. A biopsy of the skin showed neoplastic round cells infiltrating the dermis, epidermis, and follicular epithelium. The cells were round with a single large central nucleus and a moderate amount of basophilic cytoplasm. The cells frequently formed small aggregates or microabscesses within the epidermis. Neoplastic cells were positive for CD3 on immunohistochemistry. Based on this description, what is your diagnosis for this patient?

ii. Three forms of this disease exist in dogs. What are they?

iii. In most cases, diagnosis of this disease is uncomplicated based on biopsy and immunohistochemistry results (when performed). At times, however, particularly in the earlier phases of disease, diagnosis might not be quite as concrete. What other options are available for testing to confirm a diagnostic suspicion?

123 Ketoconazole, itraconazole, fluconazole, and terbinafine are antifungal drugs commonly used in veterinary dermatology to treat superficial to deep fungal diseases or yeast infections. For each drug, what is the mechanism of action?

122 i. Cutaneous epitheliotropic T-cell lymphoma.
ii. Mycosis fungoides, pagetoid reticulosis, Sézary syndrome. Clinically, mycosis fungoides cannot be distinguished from pagetoid reticulosis; the difference is based on histopathologic evaluation. In either case, the disease is generalized with localized cases reported far less frequently. Sézary syndrome is a form in which neoplastic lymphocytes are also found in peripheral lymph nodes and peripheral blood. Although lesions clinically are identical, extracutaneous neoplastic lymphocytes are not noted with the other two forms. Since all three forms appear clinically identical in dogs, the disease might be better classified with regard to subtype based on appearance: exfoliative erythroderma, plaques/nodules, ulcerative disease of the oral mucosa, and mucocutaneous forms.
iii. One option is to take advantage of the fact that clonality (expansion of neoplastic cells from the same clonal population of cells) is a hallmark of malignancy; heterogeneity of cells implies reactivity as opposed to malignancy. Canine lymphoma and other lymphoid neoplasias can be diagnosed based on the detection of clonal rearrangements of antigen receptor genes, specifically the T-cell receptor genes (CD3 region). A PCR assay has been developed to identify gene rearrangements for the specific lymphoid neoplasia (immunoglobulin rearrangement for B-cell leukemias and T-cell receptor gene rearrangements in T-cell leukemia lymphoma). A recent study identified increased expression of retinoic acid receptors and retinoid X receptors via immunohistochemistry from lymphoma tissue, whereas non-neoplastic lymphoid tissue did not show the same increased level of expression. This finding may also help differentiate lymphoma from other lymphoproliferative disease.

123 Ketoconazole, itraconazole, and fluconazole are azole antibiotics. Their mechanism of action is to inhibit cytochrome P450 and the conversion of lanosterol to ergosterol, causing accumulation of C14 methylated steroids. They also inhibit intracellular triglyceride and phospholipid biosynthesis, cell wall chitin synthesis, and oxidative and peroxidative enzymes. Terbinafine is an allylamine antifungal drug that inhibits fungal growth by disrupting sterol biosynthesis. It inhibits the formation of ergosterol by inhibiting squalene epoxidase, the enzyme responsible for converting squalene to an ergosterol precursor. Deficiency of ergosterol compromises cell wall integrity and results in impaired growth and/or death of the fungal pathogen. In mammals, biosynthesis of cholesterol uses the same squalene epoxidase; however, terbinafine shows a markedly lower binding affinity for mammalian enzymes.

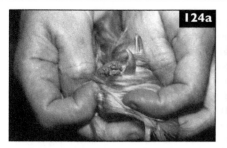

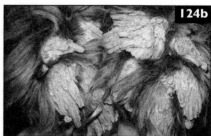

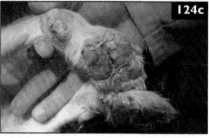

124 Foot pad hyperkeratosis is a common dermatologic problem or complaint. In addition to the history and general physical examination, careful examination of the hyperkeratosis can help narrow the differential diagnosis.

i. This dog (**124a**) is otherwise healthy. The lesions seen are present on all paws. What is the most likely differential diagnosis, and what other clinical signs could be present to support the working diagnosis?

ii. This dog (**124b**) is 7 years old and the primary complaints are 'slowing down' and 'reluctance to move quickly'. The owners report that the dog had been normal until approximately 9 months ago. The dog's heart rate, respiration, and body temperature are within normal limits. The medical record reveals a 20% increase in body weight over the last year. The hyperkeratosis is limited to the foot pads. Exudation and odor are absent. What are possible differential diagnoses?

iii. This dog (**124c**) is 10 years old and the primary complaint was lameness. In addition, physical examination revealed weight loss and the owner confirmed that the dog had been depressed and anorectic for the last several weeks. What are likely differential diagnoses?

125 Most active ingredients in shampoos remain constant despite reformulations and renaming of veterinary products. Tailoring treatment recommendations for a specific patient or disease requires a thorough understanding of the active ingredients.

i. With regard to antibacterial antiseptics, what ingredients are options?

ii. What recommendations for antipruritic therapy may be used when infections are absent?

124 i. The lesion shown is classic digital hyperkeratosis. This is common in dogs with disorders of keratinization, particularly cocker spaniel dogs. The nose should be examined to look for concurrent nasal hyperkeratosis. Hyperkeratosis around the mammae presenting as 'fronds' is a common concurrent clinical finding.

ii. The most likely are those that involve an underlying medical disease. Musculoskeletal pain can change a dog's gait and lead to abnormal foot pad keratinization. In this case there are long fronds of keratin on the foot pads growing in all directions. The lack of exudation and odor make immune-mediated diseases or infection less likely. The vague history of decreased activity and weight gain makes hypothyroidism suspect. Foot pad changes are also common in dogs with hepatocutaneous syndrome. Other possible causes include vitamin A-responsive skin disease, fatty acid deficiency, and zinc-responsive skin disease.

iii. Include, but are not limited to: immune-mediated diseases (pemphigus complex), metabolic (hepatocutaneous syndrome), severe irritant reaction, infection (bacterial or fungal), or possibly demodicosis. In most cases of primary bacterial or demodectic pododermatitis there is more exudation and swelling and less hyperkeratosis. Severe dermatophyte infection with *M. gypseum* can cause severe pedal dermatitis, but would not account for the weight loss and signs of systemic illness. These foot pads are representative of the hyperkeratosis and fissuring seen in cases of hepatocutaneous syndrome.

125 i. Common ingredients include chlorhexidine, benzoyl peroxide, acetic acid/boric acid, tris-EDTA, ethyl lactate. All of these ingredients are antiseptics, meaning their intrinsic properties allow for killing of microbial organisms. Several recent studies have evaluated the efficacy of these various antimicrobials. Two studies found chlorhexidine to be most effective when compared with other topical antimicrobials including benzoyl peroxide. Another study found *in-vitro* efficacy of acetic and boric acids to be very low.

ii. If the patient is historically prone to infection development, bathing with antiseptic shampoos should still be part of the long-term management protocol. One study evaluated the effects of conventional shampooing versus whirlpool therapy, with and without shampoo; the study showed decreased pruritus scores in patients treated with whirlpooling regardless of whether shampoo was used or not. This demonstrates the inherent benefits of topical therapy in dogs. Another study evaluated the efficacy of using ultrapure soft water with shampoo for controlling pruritus; dogs treated showed improvement in TEWL, indicating improved skin barrier recovery. In one patient who was intensely pruritic post bathing with tap water, when the same shampoo was used with well water or distilled water the dog was not pruritic. Anecdotally, colloidal oatmeal and pramoxine may be beneficial for pruritus; shampoo therapy tends to provide short-term relief to pruritic patients. Longer relief may occur if these ingredients are incorporated into leave-on lotions or conditioners.

126 A 9-year-old female spayed black dog presented for a 6-month history of non-pruritic nodular skin disease that had not responded to previous anti-biotic administration or topical bathing. The owner reported that the lesions had primarily affected the muzzle, dorsal head, and various other regions of the dog's body on haired surfaces (**126a**). Nodules were not exudative but were alopecic, variably sized, and erythematous.

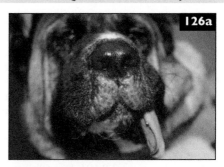
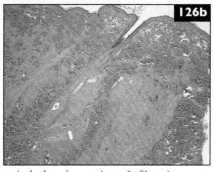

i. What are the differentials and recommended diagnostic tests?

ii. Histopathology from one of the nodules is shown (**126b**). The dermato-pathology report identified a nodular to diffuse infiltration of primarily histiocytes, small lymphocytes, and neutrophils extending through the middle dermis and subcutis. Lesions typically tracked along adnexal structures to the superficial dermis in a linear/tubular formation. Infiltration was frequently centered on blood vessels, but was only minimally vasoinvasive. No organisms were identified on special stains. Based on this report, what is the diagnosis for this patient?

iii. What treatment options should be considered for this patient?

iv. How would you counsel the owner regarding the prognosis?

127 Note the lesion shown on this cat's face (**127**). The owner reports a slow onset of the lesion and a lack of pruritus. This is an indoor/outdoor cat of unknown age. How would you work up this case?

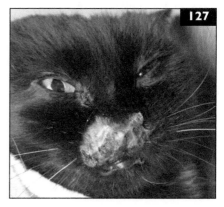

126 i. Infectious (actinomycosis, nocardiosis, bacterial pseudomycetoma, opportunistic mycobacterial infection, dermatophytic kerion, blastomycosis, histoplasmosis, coccidioidomycosis, cryptococcosis, sporotrichosis, other opportunistic fungal infection, pythiosis, lagenidiosis, prototheosis, leishmaniasis); inflammatory (sterile granuloma and pyogranuloma syndrome, reactive histiocytosis, cutaneous xanthoma, canine sarcoidosis); neoplasia (cutaneous T-cell lymphoma, mast cell tumor, metastatic neoplasia). The most important diagnostics include skin biopsy with special stains and bacterial culture for aerobic and atypical bacterial organisms such as *Mycobacterium*, *Nocardia*, and *Actinomyces* spp. Additional diagnostic testing should include CBC, serum biochemistry, urinalysis, thoracic radiographs, and CT/MRI depending on findings.

ii. Reactive histiocytosis.

iii. For solitary lesions, surgical excision is successful; however, this does not prevent development of new lesions. Topical corticosteroids may be used for localized disease. For widespread nodules, tetracycline/doxycycline and niacinamide is often effective. It may be administered alone or combined with vitamin E and fatty acid supplementation. Response to corticosteroid administration is variable, but may be as high as 50% in cases with the cutaneous form of disease. In more refractory cases, cyclosporine (modified) or leflunomide can be effective. Immunosuppressive dosing is recommended (initially) and then tapered to the lowest effective dose.

iv. Although the disease typically does not progress (e.g. the cutaneous form does not become systemic), the prognosis for durable remission is guarded. This is due to the waxing and waning nature of the disease and need for long-term treatment. If tetracycline/doxycycline and niacinamide is successful, side-effects may be minimal long term, lending to a more favorable prognosis.

127 Wear gloves when handling this patient as many of the possible differential diagnoses are zoonotic. Key initial diagnostic tests include: skin scrapings, hair pluckings, impression smears, Wood's lamp examination, and bacterial culture and sensitivity. Slow-onset lesions can be neoplastic and a skin biopsy is indicated. Medical diagnostics should include screening for FeLV and FIV since the cat goes outside. This cat proved to be FeLV and FIV positive. *D. cati* mites were found at the lesion site and from hair trichograms distant to the lesion. Skin biopsy and special stains ruled out neoplasia and microbial infections. Except for finding *Demodex* mites on the biopsy, the only other significant finding was supportive infection. Bacterial culture revealed a methicillin-resistant SIG. This was an unexpected finding since the cat had no prior history of antibiotic therapy. Treatment with topical mupirocin ointment and oral milbemycin for demodicosis resulted in marked improvement but not resolution of the lesion.

128 A 10-year-old female spayed DSH cat presented for a non-pruritic cutaneous lesion on the dorsal cervical region. The owner had noted the lesion while she was petting the cat a few days prior to examination. The cat did not seem to be bothered by the lesion; there was no evidence of pruritus or self-induced alopecia. No evidence of systemic illness was reported by the owner. On closer examination, there were three small (1–2 mm diameter) plaque-like papules present on the dorsal neck near the base of the skull. The masses were discrete, firm, and tan in appearance. The surface was alopecic; however, broad hair loss was not present surrounding the masses.

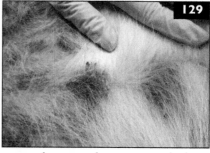

i. Cytology from an aspirate of the masses is shown (**128**). What is the diagnosis for this patient?
ii. How are these masses classified in cats with regard to histologic interpretation?
iii. What is the typical biological behavior of these cutaneous masses in cats?

129 A 7-year-old female spayed German shepherd dog was presented for recurrent skin infections over approximately the last 8 months. According to the owners, the dog had no history of skin disease prior to this. Pruritus was noted to be mild to moderate and primarily focused on the ventral abdomen where lesions were noted (**129**). The owners reported that several courses of antibiotics had been administered along with different shampoos; however, the treatments had not resolved the lesions. Otherwise, the dog seemed overall in good general health. She had gained weight (total of 2.7 kg [6 lb]) over the past 8 months and seemed less energetic; however, the owners attributed this to her age.

i. Based on the history provided by the owners, what dermatologic diagnostics should be performed?
ii. What are a few possible reasons for the recurrent skin infections in this patient?
iii. What additional diagnostics may be considered?
iv. With regard to this patient, what treatment recommendations would you make?

128 i. Mast cell tumor (MCT).

ii. As mastocytic or atypical poorly granulated MCTs. The mastocytic type is subclassified as well-differentiated or pleomorphic. Prognostic indicators are not as well defined for feline cutaneous MCTs as they have been for dogs. A recent study evaluated potential markers to determine their prognostic value for feline cutaneous MCTs. It was determined that multiple masses, pleomorphic phenotype, and high mitotic index all correlated with an unfavorable outcome. Immunohistochemistry factors including KIT (CD117) expression, telomerase expression, and proliferation index (MIB-1/Ki67 index) were also evaluated. Increased KIT immunoreactivity and Ki67 index also was associated with increased morbidity. A previous study also identified KIT expression to be potentially helpful in identifying mast cell origin; however, there did not appear to be a difference in KIT expression and MCT phenotype. Further evaluation is warranted.

iii. In general, most feline cutaneous MCTs are considered to be benign neoplasms with a low rate of local recurrence. The presence of multiple cutaneous MCTs has been associated with decreased overall survival time compared with cats with solitary masses. Involvement of regional lymph nodes or spleen is also associated with more severe disease. Solitary cutaneous MCTs without lymph node involvement typically present as benign disease with a relatively extended survival time. Median survival time is markedly decreased in cats with multiple cutaneous masses, evidence of tumor recurrence following surgical removal, and/or lymph node or splenic involvement. The prognosis is guarded for these animals.

129 i. Skin scrapings, skin cytology, possible dermatophyte culture, bacterial culture and susceptibility.

ii. (1) Bacterial resistance; (2) underlying illness leading to secondary bacterial infections: possibilities include any metabolic (renal insufficiency, hepatic disease), endocrine (hypothyroidism, hyperadrenocorticism), or neoplastic process.

iii. CBC, serum biochemistries, urinalysis.

iv. Treatment of the infection should be two-fold. If the owners are willing and able, topical control should be initiated with an antiseptic shampoo. Chlorhexidine would be a good agent to use, either alone or in combination with other antiseptics (e.g. phytosphingosine, miconazole or ketoconazole if yeast are also noted on cytology, or tris-EDTA). To get good contact with the skin, it may be beneficial to clip the hair coat short as this dog's coat is rather dense; good penetration through the fur may not be possible. Based on the results of culture and susceptibility, if an appropriate antibiotic can be used, it should be prescribed for a minimum of 3–4 weeks. The typical recommendation is to treat at least 1 week past the point of clinical resolution. This takes a minimum of 3 weeks for superficial skin infections and may take longer. With the growing prevalence of bacterial resistance, antibiotic choices are often limited.

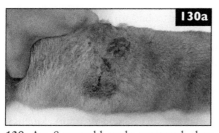

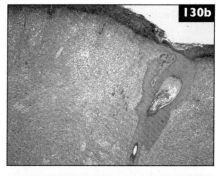

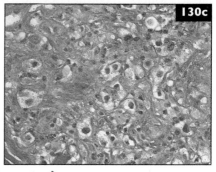

130 An 8-year-old male castrated shar pei dog presented for a 2-month history of progressive skin lesions. Initially, the dog had a swollen, thickened and erythematous lesion over the left hindlimb; the lesion measured approximately 9 cm in diameter and extended over the tarsus (130a). More recently, the lesion had grown in size and had a sticky, viscous exudate on the ulcerated surface. Additional lesions had also developed over the trunk, medial thighs, and head. Mild pruritus was evident and the dog was non-weight bearing on the left hindlimb.

i. What is the most likely explanation for the sticky, viscous exudate noted by the owners?

ii. Histologic findings from a skin biopsy of the mass are shown (130b, c). Histopathologic interpretation showed a poorly demarcated, non-encapsulated, invasive neoplastic mass extending through the entire dermis. The mass was composed of closely to widely spaced round cells in sheets; the cells had variably distinct borders and moderate to large amounts of cytoplasm. Smaller cells contained fine basophilic granules; most cells were larger with wispy and vesiculated cytoplasm. Nuclei were round to oval with multiple nucleoli. Mitotic index was high. Lymphatics were dilated with neoplastic cells. Several eosinophils were admixed with neoplastic cells. Given the description, what special stain is recommended to confirm the diagnosis?

iii. Uncontrolled cellular proliferation is a key feature of neoplasia. Measurements of cellular proliferation have been used in human and veterinary medicine to predict behaviors of tumors. What proliferation markers have been evaluated for this canine neoplasia?

131 What is phytosphingosine?

130 i. Mucin. Cutaneous mucinosis is considered to be 'normal' in the shar pei breed.

ii. MCT (grade III based on the cellular and nuclear morphology). Toluidine blue stain would better identify mast cell granules.

iii. In veterinary medicine, proliferation markers that have been evaluated for canine MCTs include staining for argyrophilic nucleolar organizer regions (AgNORs) and immunohistochemistry for proliferating cell nuclear antigen (PCNA) and Ki67. AgNORs are widely used as a measurement of tumor kinetics and metabolic activity; they identify areas in the nucleus associated with proteins and ribosomal RNA transcription. Higher AgNOR counts are associated with increased mortality, local recurrence, and metastasis for canine MCTs. PCNA interacts with DNA polymerases and has maximal expression during the synthesis phase of the cell cycle. Although studies have shown association between PCNA expression and increased mortality in canine MCTs, expression has not been proven as a prognostic indicator independent of histologic tumor grade (i.e. higher grade tumors have a tendency towards increased PCNA expression by default [increased mitotic index etc.]). Ki67 is a nuclear protein; it is expressed in all phases of the active cell cycle; however, inactive cells do not express this protein. Cells positive for Ki67 are actively involved in the cell cycle (known as the growth fraction) and are considered to be a measure of proliferation. For canine MCTs, increased Ki67 expression is associated with increased mortality, rate of local recurrence, and metastasis. KIT (also known as CD117) is a stem cell factor receptor associated with MCT development in dogs. It is encoded by the proto-oncogene c-kit. Expression of KIT has been associated with histologic grade of MCTs; increased KIT expression is noted with higher grade tumors along with increased expression of Ki67 and AgNORs.

131 A plant-based sphingosine molecule. Sphingosines are incorporated into the intercellular lipid bilayer that forms the epidermal barrier of the stratum corneum by forming ceramides. Newer shampoos and ear cleaners incorporate phytosphingosine into their products. These products may be beneficial for seborrheic skin conditions (keratoplastic function) and may improve barrier function with regard to 'normalizing' the epidermis. Claims have also been made for mild antimicrobial and antipruritic actions; this may be due to the improvement in barrier function.

132 A 6-year-old female spayed bassett hound dog presented for evaluation of chronic and recurrent bilateral ear infections of at least 8 months' duration. Previous treatments with topical and systemic medications did not resolve the clinical signs. The dog had moderate otic pruritus on physical examination and vocalized loudly when the ears were manipulated. Otoscopic examination revealed a large amount of green malodorous purulent exudate with visible ulceration along the length of the canal. Cytology from both ears showed large numbers of mixed bacterial organisms (primarily rods with large numbers of cocci admixed) and neutrophils.
i. What are possible reasons for the persistence of the bacterial ear infection?
ii. CT identified fluid opacity in both tympanic bullae. Myringotomy and canal irrigation were performed. Culture was obtained prior to irrigation; results and susceptibility profile are shown:

Antibiotic	Pseudomonas aeruginosa (strain 1)	Pseudomonas aeruginosa (strain 2)	Enterococcus spp.
Concentration (mg/ml) and susceptibility			
Penicillin G			2 S
Piperacillin	<8 S	<8 S	
Piperacillin/tazobactam	<8 S	<8 S	
Ticarcillin	<16 S	<16 S	
Ticarcillin/clavulanate	<16 S	<16 S	
Cefotaxime	>64 R	32 I	
Ceftazidime	<8 S	<8 S	
Amikacin	32 I	8 S	
Gentamicin	8 I	S S	
Tobramycin	4 S	4 S	
Ciprofloxacin	>4 R	<0.5 S	I S
Aztreonam	<8 S		
Cefepime	8 S	<4 S	
Ceftizoxime	64 R	128 R	
Imipenem	<4 S	<4 S	
Ofloxacin	>8 R	<1 S	
Cefpodoxime	>8 R	>8 R	
Levofloxacin	>8 R	<1 S	<=1 S
Rifampin			>=4 R
R = resistant; S = susceptible; I = intermediate susceptibility			

What type of organism is *Pseudomonas* spp.?
iii. What is the general susceptibility of *Enterococcus* spp. to cephalosporin antibiotics?
iv. What recommendations for management should be considered?

132 i. Occlusion, resistant organism, middle ear disease. Occlusion may be due to the presence of a mass (benign, neoplastic) or stenosis of the canal (excessive proliferation, swelling and edema, 'normal' conformation of the breed). Resistant organisms commonly encountered include multidrug-resistant *Pseudomonas* spp. or methicillin-resistant *Staphylococcus* spp. Otitis media may be caused by a mass proximal to the tympanic membrane or infection in the tympanic bulla. Sterile processes such as primary secretory otitis media may contribute to middle ear involvement; noted most commonly in Cavalier King Charles spaniel dogs.

ii. A gram-negative rod-shaped bacterial organism, found ubiquitously in nature. *Pseudomonas* spp. have been associated with severe otitis externa in dogs. *Pseudomonas* otitis can persist and recur for a variety of reasons including antimicrobial resistance, multiple strains of *Pseudomonas* with varying susceptibility profiles, and the influence of other factors such as occlusion, otitis media, or underlying inflammatory skin and ear disease. *Pseudomonas* isolates from the ears of dogs are frequently resistant to a variety of antibiotic agents. Fluoroquinolone resistance is noted commonly, especially in patients with chronic disease. When culture and susceptibility reveals mixed bacterial infection, treatment can be challenging.

iii. Intrinsically resistant.

iv. Because of the presence of both otitis externa and otitis media, topical and systemic treatment is recommended. Treatment needs to be based on the susceptibility profile of the organisms involved in the infection. Of the antibiotics evaluated, only injectable options are available to which all organisms are susceptible. Various options exist regarding topical treatment. Although ones listed as 'resistant' would not be recommended, those listed with 'intermediate' susceptibility would still be a viable option. A significantly higher MIC can be achieved in local tissues compared with serum. Continued irrigation of the canal with an antiseptic ear cleaner is recommended to inhibit microbial growth. Products containing tris-EDTA are typically beneficial in gram-negative infections, which require calcium and magnesium for formation of a viable bacterial cell wall. Given the highly resistant nature of this infection, the owner should be instructed to wear gloves when manipulating and treating the ear canals, especially if open wounds are present. Although additional investigation with regard to efficacy is necessary, bacteriophage therapy may be a viable treatment option to avoid further complications of resistance development.

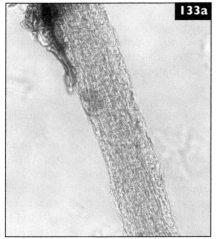

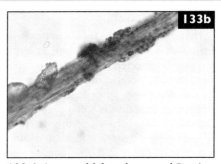

133 A 1-year-old female spayed Persian cat is presented for diffuse alopecia and excessive scaling. The owner states that 'this absolutely is NOT ringworm' because she knows what ringworm looks like and the condition did not respond to two lime sulfur dip applications. Also, none of the other seven cats or four dogs appear to have any dermatologic abnormalities.

i. You obtain a sample for a trichogram and this is observed (133a). What is your diagnosis?

ii. On examining a cytology sample, you find this (133b). Describe the abnormalities seen on the sample.

iii. What is known about the disease in this breed of cat?

134 Various options exist for the administration of ASIT. These include conventional subcutaneous injectable immunotherapy, sublingual immunotherapy, and mucosal (intranasal) immunotherapy; the latter has been evaluated for the treatment of feline experimental asthma. Currently, there is no standardized protocol for immunotherapy administration. Frequency of administration, volume, and induction protocols differ greatly between practitioners.

i. What is rush immunotherapy?

ii. In what diseases and species has rush immunotherapy been evaluated?

iii. What potential side-effects are associated with this type of immunotherapy administration? What is the general recommendation for administration when this option is pursued?

133 i. Dermatophytosis.

ii. There are numerous fungal hyphae elements visible within the hair shaft, causing distortion of the normal architecture; this leads to weakening of the hair shaft, making the infected hairs prone to breakage. This manifests clinically as alopecia. The round structures on the outside of the hair shaft are ectothrix spores. These are the infective agents of dermatophytosis.

iii. Persian cats appear to be predisposed to the development of dermatophytosis. Compared with other cat breeds, Persian cats will frequently become severely infected with a generalized form of the disease and many will remain chronically culture positive for *Microsporum canis* either due to an inability to mount effective cell-mediated immunity and/or because they are fomite carriers. These cats can appear clinically normal, making them a source of exposure to other cats, susceptible animals, and/or people. It is uncertain whether this breed predisposition is due to a genetic anomaly or other underlying factors. A similar finding has been reported in Yorkshire terrier dogs, another breed that appears predisposed to be chronically culture positive for *M. canis*. Jack Russell terriers have anecdotally been reported to be predisposed to *Trichophyton* spp. infections.

134 i. Abbreviated course of allergen administration. It has been utilized most frequently with immunotherapy injections; however, intranasal rush immunotherapy has also been studied. The induction period is shortened to one to several days compared with the normal several weeks. Gradually increasing amounts of allergen are administered, as with standard induction, but typically with fewer levels or gradations (i.e. fewer injections administered during rush versus standard induction).

ii. It is used in people with certain allergic diseases and considered to be safe and effective. In dogs it has been evaluated for the treatment of AD and found to be effective. Rush immunotherapy has been evaluated for the treatment of both asthma and AD in cats.

iii. Increased pruritus at the site of injection, urticaria and angioedema, and anaphylaxis. Because of the accelerated induction administration, side-effects tend to be more common with rush immunotherapy, therefore it is recommended that rush induction is performed in a hospital setting under close monitoring so that any adverse reactions can be identified and addressed immediately. Rush immunotherapy may be beneficial for clients who are not able to administer injections frequently (e.g. incapable or unwilling to administer every-other-day injections) or where time is a factor.

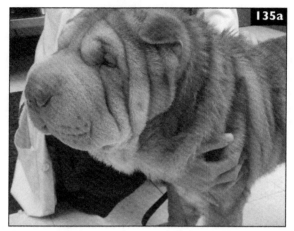

135 Shar pei dogs originated in China and for years were used as guard and hunting dogs (135a). During the Cultural Revolution, dog ownership was highly taxed and the breed neared extinction until a small group of dogs were rescued in the 1970s and taken to other countries.

i. How has the breed standard been modified? What genetic abnormality has been magnified?

ii. What skin diseases are common in this breed as a result of these changes?

136 What are the major classes of compounds used for animal flea control? What are their modes of action?

135 i. Introduction into the western world resulted in strong selection for the 'wrinkled skin phenotype'. The intentional change has been a result of selecting for dogs that have increased hyaluronan (HA) deposition in the skin. Selection of dogs that retain their skin folds into adulthood has altered the phenotype to the more heavily wrinkled 'meat mouth'. The meat mouthed

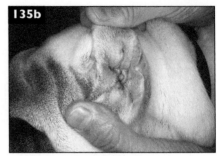

phenotypes (heavily padded muzzles) have 2–5 times higher serum levels of HA compared with other breeds and the term hyaluronanosis has been proposed as a name for this condition. HA is synthesized at the plasma membrane by three HA synthases (HAS1, HAS2, HAS3); HAS2 is the rate-limiting enzyme. It is overexpressed in dermal fibroblasts of this breed compared with other breeds, suggesting a regulatory mutation as a cause of hyaluronanosis.
ii. Clinically, these dogs seem predisposed to AD, recurrent microbial overgrowth, and demodicosis. Conditions related to excessive mucin deposition, such as chronic otitis externa (135b) due to stenotic ear canals, are common. Another common skin disease is the appearance of vesicles of varying size caused by mucin exuding from the dermis. These are easily diagnosed by gently stabbing or aspirating a lesion and noting the stringy, viscous nature of the fluid (similar to joint fluid, which also has a high concentration of HA).

136 Neonicotinoids (imidacloprid, nitenpyram, dinotefuran) act as agonists at polysynaptic nicotinic acetylcholine receptors and result in paralysis and death of adult fleas. Phenylpyrazole (fipronil) binds at the GABA-gated chloride channel causing excessive neuronal stimulation, paralysis, and death of adult fleas. Avermectins and semi-synthetic avermectins (moxidectin, selamectin) bind to receptors on glutamate-gated chloride channels leading to flaccid paralysis and death. Semicarbazone (metaflumizone) works by blocking voltage-dependent sodium channels leading to the blockage of nerve impulses causing paralysis and death. Pyrethrins and pyrethyroids work by affecting voltage-dependent sodium channels of neurons and causing paralysis. Spinosyns (spinosad, spinetoram) are non-antibacterial tetracyclic macrolides; they cause excitation of insect nervous systems leading to involuntary muscle contractions, tremors, paralysis, and death. They also have effects on GABA receptor function, which may contribute to the mechanism of action.

137 A 4-year-old female cat presented for this lesion seen on the neck (**137**). The cat was an indoor cat with no prior history of skin disease. The owners reported that the skin lesion seemed to appear suddenly; however, on further questioning the owners reported that the cat had resented petting on the head and neck for the past several weeks. At the time of admission, the lesion had been partially obscured by the hair coat and its margins and extent delineated by palpation. The lesion under the

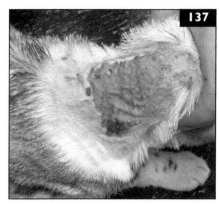

remaining hair coat felt hard, hairs were easily epilated and, although the margins of the lesion could be elevated, the crust was tightly adhered to the skin. No pain on palpation could be elicited. Clipping of the hair coat revealed the full extent of the lesion.

i. What is the medical term for the thick yellow adherent crust?
ii. What are possible differential diagnoses?

138 This dog presented with oral and mucocutaneous ulcerations (**138**).

i. What are the major immune-mediated differential diagnoses for a dog presenting with mucocutaneous ulcerations?

ii. What are the major non-immune-mediated differential diagnoses for a dog presenting with oral mucocutaneous ulcerations?

iii. The diagnosis is most often confirmed via biopsy. What is the optimum procedure for obtaining a biopsy from ulcerative lesions?

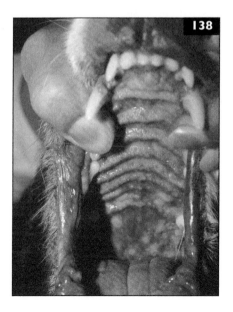

137 i. Eschar, a general term used to describe a slough of dead tissue on the surface of the skin.

ii. Differential diagnoses are difficult due to lack of information. History suggests the onset was several weeks prior to presentation; the appearance of the lesion supports that hypothesis. Strictly from the clinical appearance of the lesion, radiant thermal burn is a major differential diagnosis. These are common in cats that sit near heat stoves or fireplaces; close enough for tissue damage but far enough from immediate danger of a burn. Sun bathing in geographic regions with intense direct sunlight or repeated sleeping on electronic equipment that generates heat can also cause radiant thermal injuries of varying severity. Given the location, it is important to determine if the cat had received injections in this area or if spot-on topical flea products had been applied. Injection reactions that are irritating are likely to cause acute ulcerative lesions noticed by owners. Spot-on flea control products typically do not cause irritant reactions, but are associated with focal areas of non-inflammatory hair loss occasionally preceded by erythema. Grooming of this area is possible; if a topical caustic agent had contacted the hair coat and skin, it seems likely the cat would have been presented earlier for oral/tongue lesions. There are cases of eschar lesions in people caused by *Bartonella henselae* and rickettsial diseases post tick bite.

138 i. Bullous pemphigoid, epidermolysis bullosa acquista, pemphigus vulgaris, paraneoplastic pemphigus, EM, SLE, drug reaction, linear IgA bullous dermatosis, TEN.

ii. Renal failure should be ruled out at the time of presentation. Irritant reactions can cause oral ulceration; this can often be determined from the history or pattern of the ulcerations. Foreign body reaction (e.g. mechanical removal of plant material [burrs] from hair coat by chewing) can cause oral ulceration. It is important to rule out infectious causes of oral ulceration (e.g. viral, candidiasis); oral ulceration due to infection is rare and the host is likely to be immunocompromised.

iii. If oral ulcerations are present, it is important to look for intact vesicles and/or bullae; these are the primary lesions that lead to ulcerations. If vesicles are small, they can be harvested with a large skin biopsy punch (>6 mm); however, care must be taken not to rupture the lesion. If bullae are present, these lesions can be collected via elliptical incision. If no primary lesions can be found, an elliptical incision that extends from 'normal' to 'ulcerated' tissue should be submitted. The most valuable area of the biopsy will be the junctional area between the ulcer and 'normal' tissue.

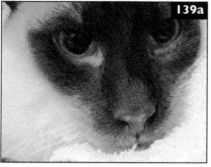

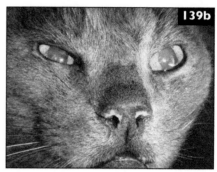

139 Note the nasal depigmentation in both of these cats (139a, b). What are possible differential diagnoses?

140 A 10-year-old female spayed shih tzu dog presented for non-healing wounds and draining tracts over the dorsum. The owner had noted the matting of the hair coat approximately 1 week ago and assumed that the dog needed to be groomed. The dog had no history of prior skin disease. On examination, there was a thick, dried purulent exudate on the dorsum, with matted hair within the crusts. When the crusts were lifted, the skin beneath was eroded and fresh exudation was present. The dog was notably painful when the skin was palpated. The hair coat was clipped; multiple draining lesions were seen once the matted hair and crusts were removed (140). The owner also reported that the dog has been coughing

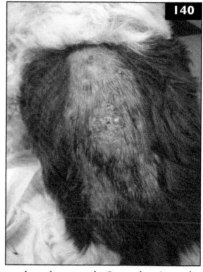

for the past week and her appetite was somewhat decreased. On palpation, the submandibular, prescapular, and popliteal lymph nodes are approximately three times larger than they should be bilaterally.

i. What diagnostics do you recommend for this patient?

ii. What are your differential diagnoses with regard to the draining lesions on the dorsum of this dog?

139 The number of differential diagnoses is limited because depigmentation is not a common skin problem in cats. Any inflammatory reaction that damages the epidermis and basal cells containing melanocytes can lead to depigmentation. In general, depigmentation can result from glucocorticoids, inflammation (although hyperpigmentation is more common), post trauma, neoplasia, immune-mediated diseases, or leuko-

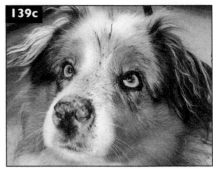

derma (congenital, hereditary). Depigmentation has been reported in association with rhinitis in cats. Close inspection of the nose in both cats reveals a lack of active inflammation, making it difficult to identify the underlying cause. Depigmentation of the nose is a hallmark of lupus; however, cutaneous lupus is still not well documented in cats. Vitiligo has been reported as a breed-associated disease in Siamese cats. Nasal depigmentation in dogs can be a sign of lupus; however, inflammation is typically present (**139c**).

140 i. Deep skin scraping, cytology, and culture and susceptibility are recommended. Skin biopsy may be indicated depending on the results of these initial diagnostics. In general, draining tracts are indicative of a deep, infiltrative disease process (e.g. deep bacterial infection, fungal infection, sterile inflammatory response, neoplasia). When draining tracts or nodules are present in any patient with skin disease, skin biopsy is recommended along with culture and susceptibility. For this patient, a CBC, serum biochemistry, and urinalysis are indicated because of the presence of systemic signs. The peripheral lymph nodes should be aspirated and thoracic radiographs considered because of the owner's report of coughing.

ii. The presence of draining tracts indicates a deep, infiltrative disease process involving the skin. Differential diagnoses include infection (deep bacterial infection including atypical infection [mycobacterial, nocardiosis, actinomycosis]; fungal infection including blastomycosis, coccidioidomycosis, histoplasmosis, sporotrichosis, opportunistic fungal disease and/or kerion reaction), inflammatory conditions (sterile granuloma/pyogranuloma syndrome, sterile nodular panniculitis, SLE, vasculitis), and neoplasia (MCT, cutaneous lymphoma, metastatic neoplasia). Depending on the history, drug eruption, topical irritant reaction, post-grooming furunculosis, and thermal burn should also be considered. In this case, skin scrapings revealed *Demodex canis* mites. This was a case of adult-onset generalized demodicosis secondary to lymphoma.

141 A 4-year-old female spayed boxer dog is presented for a mass on the medial aspect of the right pinna (141a).
i. What are your differential diagnoses for the lesion?
ii. Histopathologic examination of the mass showed 'multiple long papillary projections covered by a massive

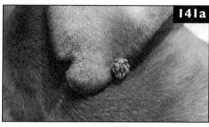

amount of partially parakeratotic scale crust. The epithelial cells covering the papillae are markedly hyperplastic and exhibit normal maturation. Occasional ballooning regeneration is present in the basal cell layer. Many of the cells have pale blue cytoplasm and occasional koilocytes with cytoplasmic clearing are evident. Cells rarely contain pale basophilic intranuclear inclusion bodies'. What is the diagnosis based on the clinical signs and histologic findings?
iii. This disease has several forms or clinical syndromes in the dog. Describe them.

142 A 5-year-old female spayed mixed-breed dog presents with an acute onset of skin lesions. Lesions developed in the third week of cephalexin treatment for a bacterial pyoderma. Small 1–2 mm erosions/ulcers are symmetrically distributed on the hard palate and on the lips. Skin lesions are most severe on the ventral abdomen. Numerous and coalescing, polycyclic rings of erythema are diffusely distributed on the ventral

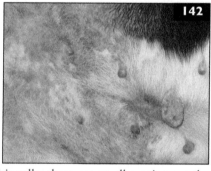

thorax, abdomen, and flanks (142). Additionally, there are small erosions at the mucocutaneous junction of several mammae and the anal ring. A skin tag on the ventral chest is not affected. There are no findings suggestive of internal disease. In addition to the cephalexin, the dog received chlorhexidine shampoo, an oral ivermectin-based heartworm preventive and a topical imidacloprid-containing flea preventive administered 21 days ago. Results of a CBC and serum chemistries are within normal range. A skin biopsy of several erythematous rings shows cell-poor interface dermatitis with multiple apoptotic keratinocytes in all cell layers of the epidermis, satellitosis, and parakeratotic hyperkeratosis.
i. Based on the historical, clinical, and histopathologic findings, what is the most likely diagnosis?
ii. What in the history is compatible with your likely diagnosis?
iii. How would you treat this dog?

141 i. Exophytic viral papilloma, non-viral squamous papilloma.

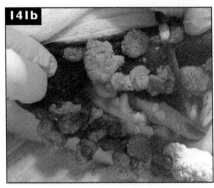

ii. Exophytic viral papilloma.
iii. Oral papillomatosis (141b) is usually a self-limiting but contagious viral disease; however, lesions may persist or progress to other body regions. Ocular papillomas are related to oral papillomas, and are considerably less common. Lesions typically are confined to the conjunctiva, cornea, and eyelid margins. Canine genital papilloma is presumed to be similar to oral papillomatosis because the lesions are contagious. Cutaneous papillomas are typically solitary lesions induced by a subtype of papillomavirus. These masses are caused by a papillomavirus that is different from the virus which causes oral papillomatosis in the dog. Lesions are most common in dogs <2 years of age, but they can occur in any age dog. Cutaneous inverted papilloma is a rare endophytic variant of the more common cutaneous exophytic papilloma. Multiple papillomas of the foot pad are found primarily in adult dogs; however, it is not confirmed if lesions are due to a papilloma virus. Papillomavirus-associated pigmented plaques have been described primarily in miniature schnauzer and pug dogs. This form of papillomavirus has shown potential for malignant transformation.

142 i. EM, a T lymphocyte-mediated reaction against individual keratinocytes resulting in cell death (apoptosis). EM is an uncommon idiosyncratic cutaneous reaction pattern having multiple forms of bizarre patterns of erythema with mucosal and cutaneous ulceration.
ii. Idiosyncratic drug reactions or eruptions can look like and mimic many other dermatoses. The index of suspicion is heightened based on the temporal history (timing of drug administration until observed lesions) and distribution of lesions (especially in non-haired or sparsely haired body regions including the oral cavity).
iii. Search for an underlying trigger of EM and remove it, if possible. Given the onset of clinical lesions during the prescribed course of cephalexin, this antibiotic is highly suspect. Chlorhexidine likely was not involved in the disease process because not all of the bathed skin was affected. Likewise, the use of this topical treatment likely did not cause the oral lesions. Nevertheless, it is prudent to discontinue all previously administered medications where applicable. Since this patient did not have systemic signs associated with the adverse drug reaction, no other treatments were prescribed and all the clinical lesions resolved 2 weeks after drug withdrawal.

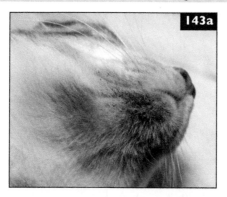

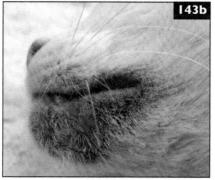

143 Feline 'chin acne' is a clinical reaction pattern in cats (**143a, b**). The number of sebaceous glands on the chin of cats is increased; territory marking is exhibited by facial rubbing on objects. Chin acne occurs when there is inflammation and plugging of hair follicles. There are a number of diagnostic approaches to feline chin acne, but one approach is similar to that of canine pyoderma: simple (acute and/or first time) or complex (chronic and/or recurrent).
i. What are the common differential diagnoses for a cat with a first time occurrence of chin acne regardless of age?
ii. What are the common differential diagnoses for a cat with chronic or recurrent episodes of chin acne regardless of age? What diagnostic tests are indicated?

144 What is the name of the biting louse of dogs found only in warm climates, and what is the name of the biting louse of cats?

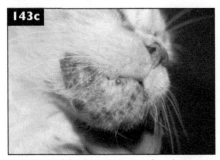

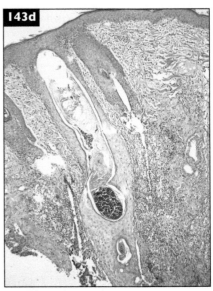

143 i. Mild plugging can be due to a mild keratinization disorder or facial rubbing. Differentials for lesions that are more extensive (**143a**) include dermatophytosis, demodicosis, *Malassezia* and/or bacterial disease, and acute dental pain.

ii. Includes chin rubbing due to pruritus from AD, food allergy, and chronic dental pain. Clinical presentation usually includes alopecia, swelling, exudation, papules, pustules, and/or furuncules (**143b**). Clinical clues that the cat may have facial pruritus or pain include blunted whiskers and skin lesions on the face and/or ears. Foreign body reactions can cause chronic chin acne, most commonly keratin from ruptured hair follicles, plant material, or insect bites (embedded stingers). Chronic recurrent chin acne can also be caused by keratinization disorders. These cats will develop lesions at a young age; lesions worsen as a result of inflammation, follicular rupture, and granulation tissue (**143c**). Skin biopsy may reveal extensive dilated comedones and furunculosis, which are difficult to treat due to the cystic nature of the lesions (**143d**). Core diagnostics (skin scraping, impression cytology, DTM fungal culture) are recommended initially. Food trials and allergy testing are needed to confirm pruritus as an underlying trigger. Biopsy may be warranted in more difficult cases.

144 *Heterodoxus spiniger* (dog louse) and *Felicola subrostratus* (cat louse).

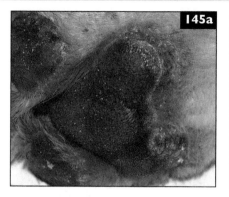

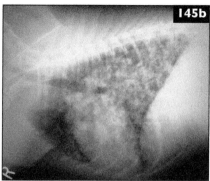

145 A 3-year-old male Labrador retriever dog from the Midwestern region of the USA was presented for the problem of lameness, depression, and cough. Examination of the dog revealed that the lameness was associated with lesions on the paws (145a). A radiograph of the thorax was obtained (145b). Cytology from purulent exudate from the margins of a paw lesion was examined (145c).

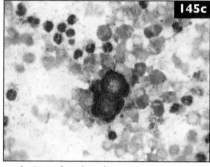

i. What is the diagnosis?
ii. What are the current treatment recommendations for this disease?
iii. Besides clinical signs, how is response to therapy monitored?

146 The ventrum of a 3-year-old mixed-breed dog that presented for the complaint of pruritus and 'scabs' is shown (146).
i. What is the name of the lesion shown (arrow)?
ii. Impression smears and bacterial cultures confirm that this is bacterial pyoderma. What is this type of pyoderma commonly referred to as?
iii. Although these lesions are classic

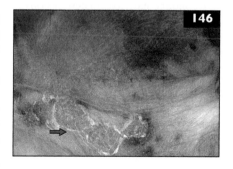

and typical of bacterial pyoderma, what other diseases need to be considered?

145 i. Fungal pneumonia due to blastomycosis with dissemination to the skin. *Blastomyces dermatitidis* is a dimorphic fungus that exists in the environment as a saprophyte; when it is inhaled it transforms into a yeast. This organism is found predominantly in North America (endemic to the Midwestern region) but has been identified in Africa, India, Europe, and Central America. Dogs used for duck and raccoon hunting are at greater risk, possibly because the organism is common near waterways, especially near beaver dams. The mode of transmission is via inhalation; dogs are more susceptible than people. This organism has low zoonotic risk; infections in both owners and dogs are considered to be coincidental exposure from the same source. However, traumatic inoculation can occur (e.g. pathologists performing necropsy of an infected host).
ii. Itraconazole is the first-line treatment for non-life-threatening systemic mycoses without CNS involvement. If there is ocular and/or CNS involvement, fluconazole is recommended (improved penetration through the blood–brain and blood–ocular barriers). A comparison of itraconazole versus fluconazole did not reveal a significant difference with respect to remission or relapse rate. Treatment with fluconaozle was longer but less expensive than with itraconazole.
iii. Treatment is monitored by urine antigen tests for blastomycosis. The sensitivity of this test is 93.5% in urine and 87.0% in serum. Treatment continues until there are two negative tests.

146 i. Epidermal collarette. This lesion is considered a 'hallmark' of bacterial pyoderma.
ii. Superficial spreading pyoderma, also known as 'exfoliative superficial pyoderma'. This is a clinical name for a superficial bacterial infection of the skin characterized by the presence of large epidermal collarettes that spread across the skin with an advancing margin consisting of a raised crust. Typically, the surrounding skin is erythematous. This is the most common form of superficial pyoderma in the dog. In long-haired dogs (e.g. collies and Shetland sheep dogs), these lesions often develop on the trunk and become large (6–10 cm in diameter), accompanied by large areas of secondary hair loss. These lesions are seen commonly in dogs with complex bacterial pyoderma, particularly in dogs with underlying AD. 'Older' textbooks referred to these lesions as 'bacterial hypersensitivity' due to their pruritic nature and occurrence in dogs with underlying pruritic diseases. The mechanism of lesion development is believed to be associated with a staphylococcal exfoliative toxin that causes loss of keratinotcyte cell–cell adhesion in the superficial epidermis. Exfoliative toxins have been identified in *Staphylococcus pseudintermedius*; injection of these toxins into mice creates characteristic skin exfoliation.
iii. PF, EM, sterile eosinophilic pustulosis, pustular dermatphytosis, demodicosis.

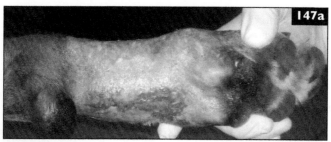

147 A 5-year-old male neutered Labrador retriever dog with an incompletely excised peripheral nerve sheath tumor of the distal limb is presented after the second week of a 4-week definitive-intent radiation therapy protocol (an attempt to sterilize the tumor field and kill any residual neoplastic cells, leading to an effective 'cure' of the nerve sheath tumor) for the problem of erythema, pruritus, and varying degrees of desquamation of the skin in the treatment field (147a). The owners are concerned about how they should be managing him at home.
i. How does progressive radiation dermatitis present in the patient?
ii. What treatment strategies are used to prevent progressive radiation dermatitis?

148 A 4-year-old male neutered Cavalier King Charles spaniel (CKCS) presents with moderate neck pain and a slight left-sided head tilt of 2 weeks' duration. The dog also 'guards' or 'protects' his neck and will occasionally spontaneously vocalize. The dog scratches his neck and ears frequently, but pruritus is absent elsewhere on the body. Recently, the owner thinks the dog has developed impaired hearing. The dog has no previous history of ear disease. Clinical examination reveals the dog to have neck pain along with a slightly diminished left-sided menace response. Mentation, cranial nerve reflexes other than menace response, postural reactions, and conscious proprioception are normal. No skin lesions are present. From gross inspection, the ears are free of odor and discharge.
i. Based on the available information, what are the possible locations of the lesion or abnormality that is causing the dog's presenting signs.
ii. Otic examination shows the epithelium to be smooth and intact with no purulent, ceruminous, or hemorrhagic discharge. No visible mass is present in either canal. The left tympanic membrane is opaque and bulging laterally into the external canal. Given the patient's signs, are there other diagnostics you would like performed?

147 i. Early radiation dermatitis manifests as erythema, pruritus, and scaly dry desquamation. Advanced radiation dermatitis manifests as moist desquamation and necrosis in extreme cases (**147b**).

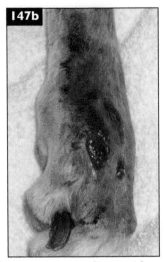

ii. There is no gold-standard approach in the prevention and management of progressive radiation dermatitis. Practice tends to be institution and site specific. Veterinary and human clinical trials have evaluated the efficacy of various treatment recommendations, but results have been mixed. As preventives, aloe vera and vitamin E topical ointments/gels, oral zinc and pentoxifylline supplementation, topical corticosteroid, and sucralfate creams are frequently prescribed. A small randomized study (20 human patients) did show statistical benefit using a topical cream containing hyaluronic acid, glycyrrhetinic acid, and anti-protease and antioxidant compounds during therapy; however, patient numbers were too small to fully evaluate the potential benefit of this therapy.

148 i. Facial nerve, cervical spine, and/or external, middle and/or inner ear.
ii. MRI of the brain, foramen magnum region, cervical neck, and bullae is indicated to exclude Chiari-like malformation/syringomyelia and primary secretory otitis media. Both of these conditions are thought to be hereditary in CKCSs. Canine Chiari-like malformation occurs when a portion of the cerebellum descends through the foramen magnum, resulting in abnormal flow and pressures in CSF. Syringomyelia is the condition caused by these dynamic changes in CSF leading to excessive cystic fluid accumulation within the spinal cord ('syrinx' formation), which can be visualized with advanced imaging modalities. Common clinical signs associated with Chiara-like malformation/syringomyelia in dogs include cervical hyperesthesia, pericervical pruritus seen as scratching, diminished menace response, facial nerve deficits, proprioceptive deficits, and seizures. Some CKCSs may remain asymptomatic in spite of documented imaging abnormalities.

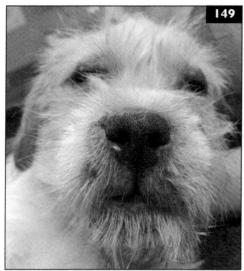

149 A 16-week-old male intact Shih tzu puppy presented with a 1-month history of progressive skin problems. Clinical signs were noted shortly following administration of the second series of vaccinations. The owner described swelling and redness, which began around both eyes and progressed to include the muzzle and chin (**149**). The dog was noted to be severely pruritic/uncomfortable to the point of causing traumatic ulcers and erosions along the affected regions. Although reported to be a quiet puppy in general, the dog also appeared to be somewhat lethargic recently. There had been no beneficial response noted to a 2-week course of oral antibiotics or a tapering anti-inflammatory course of prednisone. On physical examination, submandibular, prescapular, and popliteal lymph nodes were enlarged.
i. What are the differential diagnoses for this patient?
ii. What diagnostic recommendations should be made for this patient?
iii. Cytology of the lymph node aspirate showed suppurative inflammation without any obvious infectious organisms. Biopsy of the skin on the muzzle showed diffuse pyogranulomatous dermatitis and panniculitis. Special stains were all negative. What is the diagnosis based on this information?
iv. How is the disease treated?

150 What is PSOM?

149 i. Demodicosis, deep pyoderma, dermatophytosis, angioedema, distemper, juvenile cellulitis.
ii. Skin scrapings, impression smears of the exudates, fine needle aspirate of the lymph nodes, possible culture and susceptibility. Dermatophytosis rarely causes systemic signs and lymphadenopathy. In some cases skin biopsy may be needed to confirm the diagnosis.
iii. Juvenile cellulitis.
iv. Juvenile cellulitis is treated with immunosuppressive doses of prednisone; however, combination treatment with cyclosporine has been shown to be an effective treatment for the disease. Lack of early recognition can lead to permanent scarring. If a positive response is noted to appropriate therapy within 4–5 days of initiation, the long-term prognosis is good. In severely affected dogs, permanent scarring may be a noted consequence of the disease. Untreated, the disease can be fatal.

150 Primary secretory otitis media, a condition most commonly seen in Cavalier King Charles spaniels (CKCSs). It occurs when an excessive amount of viscous mucoid material fills the tympanic cavity, resulting in a bulging ipsilateral ear drum and neurologic abnormalities including craniocervical pain, head tilt, ataxia, facial nerve paresis/paralysis, nystagmus, and seizures. Scratching of the head/neck, with or without otitis externa, and impaired hearing are other reported signs. Mucus accumulation is thought to be secondary to poor drainage caused by a pressure mismatch resulting from uncoordinated muscular movements between the Eustachian tube and the pharynx. Removal of the mucus plug (**150**) followed by bulla flushing after myringotomy (general anesthesia required) drastically improves or resolves signs. Relapses are common, requiring repeated myringotomy and bulla content evacuation. Insertion of tympanostomy tubes to improve drainage of the bulla has been reported. MRI of the skull and neck is generally recommended in CKCSs with clinical signs possibly attributed to PSOM or Chiari-like malformation/syringomyelia since similar signs may be present with each condition. Documentation of concurrent Chiari-like malformation/syringomyelia abnormalities in a dog with PSOM is important as the patient's signs may not improve or resolve after solely removing the mucus plug from the middle ear.

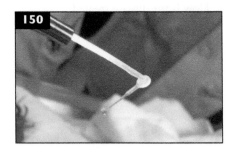

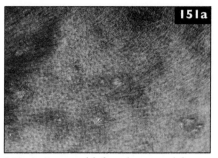 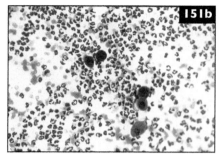

151 A 5-year-old female spayed boxer dog was presented for the complaint of lameness, depression, anorexia, and pain and exudation on the dorsum along the interscapular area. Close inspection of the skin revealed a large focal area of matting of the hair coat. After the area was clipped, a large number of intact pustules (151a) was noted. Dermatologic examination revealed crusting of the foot pads and a diffuse pustular eruption. Cytologic examination of the pustules is shown (151b). The owner reported that this was the third time the dog had developed a 'reaction' in this area post application of a spot-on flea control product. The dog had no prior history of skin disease. During the first episode the dog developed only a mild area of erythema approximately 14 days after application. After the second application, the reaction occurred much sooner (within 7 days) and was limited to a focal area. This time the lesions developed within 48 hours and the dog was febrile with a more widespread distribution of skin lesions.

i. What are the cells shown in **151b**?

ii. Bacterial culture was negative. A skin biopsy of the area revealed intracorneal pustules with large numbers of acantholytic keratinocytes. Areas of acantholysis extended into the hair follicles. Special stains were negative for any infectious agents. What is the most likely diagnosis?

152 i. What strategies are used to manage radiation dermatitis (see also case **147**)?

ii. What is the typical time course and doses at which radiation dermatitis presents?

151 i. Acantholytic keratinocytes.

ii. The most likely diagnosis is PF. In this case, the underlying trigger was a spot-on flea control product containing metaflumizone–amitraz. This product has been associated with pustular acantholytic dermatitis in dogs, suggesting a contact drug-triggered PF. In a study of metaflumizone–amitraz-associated pustular acantholytic dermatitis in 22 dogs, the authors confirmed a PF-like drug reaction at the site of flea control application.

152 i. The treatment site should be clean, dry, and protected from trauma and irritation. The site can be managed with warm water soaks or gentle washing with a mild soap and patting dry. Hydrophilic moisturizing creams provide rapid relief for early dry desquamation and minor irritation. Topical corticosteroid ointments (e.g. hydrocortisone, triamcinolone) are beneficial for pruritus, but should be discontinued if moist desquamation develops. Once moist desquamation develops, longer more frequent soaks should be used for natural debridement. Non-stick, non-occlusive, and/or hydrogel wound dressings should be used. If moist desquamation develops with >5–10 Gy remaining, debridement soaks should be continued and radiation withheld until new skin islets are visualized.

ii. Erythema is variable and closely related to radiation effects (vasodilation) on vessels. Epidermal changes are based on radiodepletion of cellular compartments with germinal and stem cells being at greatest risk of injury. Based on turnover time of canine epidermis (approximately 21 days), progression from dry to moist desquamation is seen about 2–3 weeks after starting radiotherapy. Although skin tolerance experiences a significant volume and dose rate accumulation effect, erythema and dry desquamation typically present at cumulative doses around 20–30 Gy with progression to moist desquamation around 40–50 Gy when administered in 2 Gy fractions. Epidermal appendages start to display transient loss in function early and may progress to permanent loss if doses are sufficient. After cumulative doses of about 10–12 Gy administered in 2 Gy fractions, sebaceous gland and hair follicle dysfunction is observed.

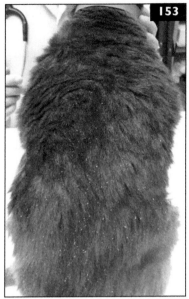

153 This 6-year-old female spayed cat was presented for the complaint of persistent scaling. The owners had adopted the cat 1 year ago. It lived indoors and there were no other pets in the household. On questioning, the owners reported a gradual development of scaling over the last year and moderate pruritus. Except for the skin lesions, physical examination was unremarkable. Dermatologic examination revealed diffuse scaling throughout the hair coat including along the ventrum and legs (**153**). Some of the hairs were pierced by scales. A small area of the hair coat was clipped and scales were adhered to the skin. No other lesions were noted. Although previously recommended at routine health visits, the owners declined flea control because the cat lived indoors.

i. Given the above information, what is the most likely clinical diagnosis?

ii. How would you confirm your clinical diagnosis?

iii. When cats are presented for an examination, increased scaling is often observed. What are possible causes?

154 What is known about the relationship between vitamin D and AD in the dog?

153 i. Superficial bacterial pyoderma with or without concurrent *Malassezia* overgrowth. Another highly suspect disease would be *Cheyletiella* spp. because of the excessive scaling and pruritus.

ii. Impression smears using glass slides and/or clear acetate tape preparations can be used to identify bacteria and yeast.

iii. Common causes are fear and stress. In the case of fear, adrenaline results in piloerection and shedding hairs and scales adjacent to the hairs and skin. If the owner reports the cat has 'dry skin' at home, fear would not explain persistent scaling in its home environment. On the other hand, many more cats with true dermatologic problems have had their scaling attributed to 'humidity or dry hair coat'. The theory is that cats spend large portions of the day sunbathing or nestled up against a heating duct and this heat results in 'dry skin'. Sunbathing and heat seeking behavior are universally present in this species, yet only a small number of cats exhibit this problem. This becomes problematic when trying to determine the time line (start of the disease) and/or seasonality. Other common causes of scaling include lack of grooming due to obesity or osteoarthritis.

154 Vitamin D is increasingly being recognized as an immune modulator in humans. Increasing evidence suggests the potential for vitamin D to inhibit Th2 responses. Furthermore, evidence suggests that vitamin D might promote cathelicidin expression on the skin; cathelicidins are important in skin defense mechanisms against microbial infections (e.g. bacterial infections). Vitamin D supplementation has been shown to provide significant improvement in lesion scores in a small group of children with winter-related AD. Further research is needed, but these findings suggest a possible role for vitamin D with regard to allergies in humans.

In dogs, there has been little work investigating the potential role for vitamin D in allergies. A recent study measured serum 25-hydroxyvitamin D [25(OH)D] concentrations in dogs receiving anti-inflammatory prednisone for the treatment of AD and compared these levels with those of healthy dogs. The dogs treated with prednisone did not have significantly different levels of 25(OH)D compared with the healthy dogs. However, dogs with a suboptimal response to prednisone were found to have significantly lower levels of 25(OH)D compared with dogs that had marked improvement. The study also compared 25(OH)D levels between dogs that responded well to cyclosporine with suboptimal responders and found no significant differences. Further studies are needed to investigate the relationship between vitamin D and response to steroids in atopic dogs and/or if it can be used as an adjuvant treatment for canine AD.

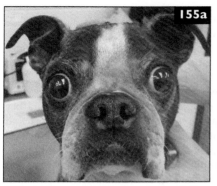 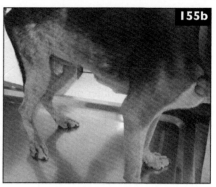

155 A 7-year-old male castrated Boston terrier dog presented for multifocal erythema and hair loss of several months' duration (155a, b). The owner also reported that the dog would frequently have episodes of exercise intolerance, fatigue, frequent panting, and near respiratory distress with noticeable inspiratory stridor. The owner also felt that the dog's head had changed from how it used to look; the eyes appeared to be bulging more than usual. On examination, the dog's skin was noted to be thin and atonic.

i. What is canine acromegaly (hypersomatotropism)?
ii. What is the typical signalment?
iii. Which of the dog's clinical signs are compatible with this diagnosis?

156 A 3-year-old female spayed Labrador retriever dog was presented with multifocal, progressive, non-pruritic areas of alopecia on the head, neck, and legs. The lesions were not specific to any particular condition and it was determined that a skin biopsy from the affected areas would likely provide the best information to identify the condition affecting this patient.

i. Which areas for biopsy should be collected from this patient?
ii. How should the skin biopsies be collected?
iii. What should be done with the collected skin biopsies?

155 i. An excess of circulating growth hormone, often caused by an increase in circulating progesterone. The disease may develop following prolonged administration of progestins, especially medroxyprogesterone acetate, or in intact older female dogs during diestrus. Rarely, acromegaly may be caused by a growth hormone-secreting tumor of the pituitary gland.
ii. Middle-aged to older intact female dogs.
iii. The most commonly reported clinical signs include inspiratory respiratory distress and stridor. This is due to the increase in soft tissue in the oropharyngeal and orolaryngeal areas. On physical examination, this patient had a severely elongated and thickened soft palate. Patients with acromegaly may also have increased body size, often noted as enlargement of the limbs, feet, head, and abdomen. In this dog's case, the broader head explained the bulging eyes noted by the owner. In typical cases the skin becomes thickened and more folded, particularly around the head, extremities, and neck. This is due to connective tissue proliferation in the dermis and deposition of hyaluronates leading to interstitial edema formation. This feature was not noted on skin biopsy from this dog; rather, epidermal atrophy was reported, a feature common to many endocrine dermatopathies.

156 i. Fully developed lesions or early developing lesions are preferred; 'older' lesions are less diagnostic.
ii. Do not shave, wash, or scrub lesions as this could remove diagnostic material. Gently clip adjacent hairs without touching the skin or removing crusts or scales. Subcutaneous injection of anesthetic is necessary unless the dog is sedated. Collect specimens from the center of lesions when using a punch biopsy. For transitional areas, use an elliptical excision that spans affected and non-affected skin; orient the ellipse parallel to hair growth. In biopsies collected from areas of alopecia, it is important to mark a line parallel to the direction of the hair growth (**156**). This helps the pathologist orient biopsies to be trimmed for histologic examination.
iii. Gently blot the specimen to remove blood and immediately place in a solution with 10% neutral buffered formalin, with the ratio of tissue to formalin at least 1:10. Punch biopsies can be placed directly in formalin; excisional biopsies must be placed on a piece of wooden tongue depressor or cardboard to avoid curling and folding of specimens. Larger punch biopsies should not be placed in a specimen mesh/cassette; this can distort specimens. Formalin only penetrates 1 cm of tissues. Specimens >1 cm should be trimmed to allow proper fixation. After fixing for 24 hours, a smaller container with less formalin can be used to submit samples.

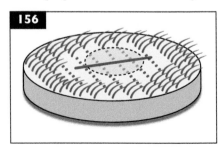

157 With regard to the dog in case **155**:
i. How is canine acromegaly diagnosed?
ii. How is the disease typically treated?

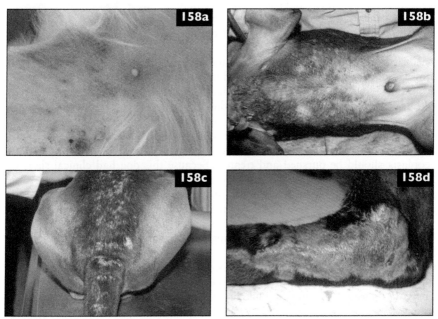

158 The term 'pyoderma' literally means 'pus in the skin'. By convention, when the term 'pyoderma' is used in veterinary dermatology it is assumed to be referring to bacterial skin infections caused by *Staphylococcus* spp. Bacterial pyoderma can be classified by a variety of schemes. One scheme is based on whether or not an underlying trigger can be identified: secondary or primary (i.e. idiopathic). Another scheme classifies the infection based on the underlying etiology (*Staphylococcus* spp., *Nocardia*). The most common scheme used in clinical practice is classification by depth of pyoderma: superficial or deep.
i. What clinical manifestations of bacterial pyoderma are demonstrated in these four images (**158a–d**)?
ii. What is difficult about the classification of intertrigo and pyotraumatic dermatitis?

Answers: 157, 158

157 i. A tentative diagnosis is made based on supportive history and clinical signs in an intact, cycling female dog. This dog did not have the expected signalment. Documentation of increased serum growth hormone is required to diagnose the condition definitively. Currently, there are no commercially available assays to detect circulating growth hormone in the dog. Increased insulin-like growth factor is consistent with a diagnosis of acromegaly and may be used as a marker of disease. An adrenal hormone panel may document increased progesterone hormone; this was elevated in this patient.

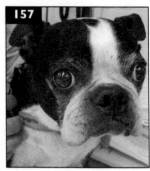

ii. In most cases where progesterone-induced acromegaly is proven or suspected, withdrawal of exogenous progestin therapy and/or ovariohysterectomy are curative. Clinical signs associated with the excess circulating growth hormone, including tissue proliferation, are typically reversible. Medical management with aglepristone is a viable treatment option. In atypical cases, work-up for pituitary neoplasia should be pursued and treated. Because this dog had clinical signs of increased growth hormone and an elevation in insulin-like growth factor and progesterone, pituitary neoplasia was suspected. The dog responded well to mitotane administration, with near complete resolution of clinical signs (**157**).

158 i. (**158a**) impetigo, (**158b**) spreading pyoderma, (**158c**) folliculitis, (**158d**) deep pyoderma.

ii. These two clinical presentations can appear clinically and/or histologically as either superficial or deep pyoderma, depending on the etiology and chronicity. Intertrigo is caused by moisture, maceration, and chronic friction from appositional areas. These lesions are often managed similarly to focal areas of superficial pyoderma. Histologically, epidermal lesions consist of severe erosion and/or ulcerations with exudation. Superficial crusts contain neutrophils and serum and are often colonized by bacteria. Necrosis may extend into the dermis and there may be mild to moderate neutrophilic or lymphoplasmacytic infiltration. Pyotraumatic dermatitis has two clinical presentations with different histologic findings: (1) epidermal lesions consisting of severe erosion, ulceration, and exudation. Superficial crusts contain degenerating neutrophils and are often colonized by gram-positive bacteria. The adjacent epidermis may be spongiotic. Necrosis and inflammation may extend into the dermis with a lymphoplasmacytic infiltrate with or without eosinophils; (2) in addition to the findings described above, deep folliculitis, follicular rupture, and diffuse inflammation in the deep dermis can also be seen. Coalescence of ruptured furuncles is a common finding. The underlying trigger for both forms of pyotraumatic dermatitis is usually a hypersensitivity reaction.

159 A cat rescue organization asked for assistance with recurrent *Otodectes* spp. infestations. The rescue facility's admission of cats was limited and based solely on space availability. During admission, cats were screened for diseases, housed in individual cages in an isolation room for 14 days, vaccinated for feline upper respiratory diseases and panleukopenia, and prophylactically administered a single application of selamectin. After this period, if room was available, cats were moved to large open floor adoption rooms

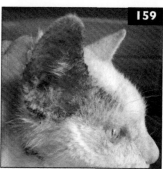

appropriately furnished for cats. If room was not available, cats remained in individual cages until such space was available. A careful investigation of the facility, the cats, and medical records revealed that *Otodectes* infestations were occurring only in rooms where cats were allowed to co-mingle. In addition, there was no evidence that cats with clinical ear mite infestations received treatment other than one application of selamectin. Clinical signs varied from typical brown-black debris to severe pruritus, as shown here (159). The rescue facility director is concerned about environmental infestation of the group housing rooms with *Otodectes* spp. What is the likelihood that cats are being reinfested from the environment?

160 A 4-month-old cat was presented for the problem of hair loss and crusting on the ears. Skin scrapings, flea combings, and ear swabs were negative for parasites. A Wood's lamp examination of hairs plucked from skin lesions revealed intrafollicular bright green fluorescence of the hair bulbs. A direct examination is shown (160). A DTM plate was inoculated via

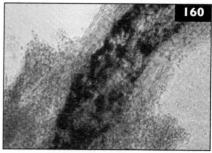

toothbrush fungal culture technique. Further questioning revealed that this was a single cat household and the cat had only been in the home for 3 days prior to presentation. Because the kitten was not yet litter box trained, the kitten was confined to a small room in the home.

i. Can you make a definitive diagnosis at this point? If so, what is it?

ii. The owner is unwilling to commit to your treatment recommendations pending confirmation of the fungal culture. What recommendations are important to make during the 7–14 day incubation period?

159 It is possible. The survival of *O. cynotis* mites off the host has been studied under both natural and laboratory conditions. At 10°C (50°F) and 95% relative humidity mites were able to survive in the laboratory for 15–17 days; however, at 34°C (93.2°F), survival was only 5–6 days. Female mites survived longer than males. In natural conditions, mites could live off the host for 12 days at temperatures ranging from 12–14°C (53.6–57.2°F) and relative humidity between 57% and 83%. Looking at both experimental and field conditions, mites can live off the host over a wide range of temperature (10–34°C [50–93.2°F]) and humidity (57–95%). Animal facilities will most likely experience a range of temperature and humidity that will allow for survival of mites off host for at least a few days. Mites and debris are most likely to collect in areas where cats sleep or frequent, making these areas 'hot spots' for transmission. In this situation, all the rooms were cleaned, disinfected, and then treated with an environmental product labeled for control of fleas. Cat beds and perching posts were cleaned or removed depending on their composition. While rooms were being treated, cats were moved to individual cages, their ears were cleaned and treated appropriately, and all were retreated with a spot-on therapy for flea control with dual efficacy against ear mites (e.g. selamectin, imidacloprid plus moxidectin).

160 i. Yes, *Microsporum canis* dermatophytosis. This is the only fungal pathogen of importance in veterinary medicine that fluoresces. The finding of fluorescing hairs alone is not diagnostic of a dermatophyte infection; however, microscopic examination of hairs and identification of ectothrix spores is definitive. Note the prominent cuffs of spores around the hair shaft. Wood's lamp examinations are most time- and cost-efficient as a screening tool when examining suspect skin lesions, especially in cats.
ii. First, pending confirmation of the culture, the owner should confine the kitten to a room that can be easily cleaned to prevent spore deposition in the environment. Spores do not proliferate in the environment, but their presence can complicate post-treatment fungal cultures and potentially be a risk factor for susceptible hosts. Second, the owner should mechanically clean the room daily and wash areas with detergent to remove infective material. Disinfectants are used to eliminate spores not removed via cleaning. Third, the owner should be encouraged to start topical therapy to minimize spread of spores in the environment. Fourth, any other health issues should be addressed (e.g. intestinal parasites, vaccinations, diet). Fifth, the owner should be instructed to use common sense and good hand hygiene after handling the kitten. Dermatophytosis is a zoonotic disease.

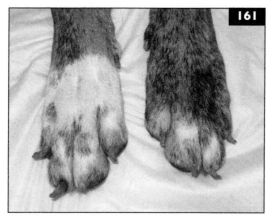

161 A 5-year-old male neutered mixed-breed dog presents for loss of nails and mild intermittent lameness. Initially the dog lost a single nail on the left front paw, but after several weeks the owners report multiple missing nails from all the paws. Clinical examination finds a generally healthy dog with problems limited to the nails. Onychorrhexis, onychodystrophy, onycholysis, onychomadesis, and onychalgia without purulent paronychia are seen from various and multiple claws/digits on each paw (161). The dog eats an over-the-counter commercial diet and receives monthly flea and heartworm prevention. No other animals are in the household.

i. Define onychorrhexis, onychodystrophy, onycholysis, onychomadesis, onychalgia, and paronychia.

ii. List some differential diagnoses for single claw abnormalities on a paw as opposed to when multiple nails from more than one paw are affected?

iii. If distal digit amputation (P3 removal) for biopsy is performed in a dog, what affected digit(s) would be the best one to remove?

iv. What is symmetrical lupoid onychodystrophy (SLO)?

162 The diagnosis of *Microsporum canis* dermatophytosis was confirmed in the cat in case 160.

i. What treatment options should now be considered?

ii. Which topical antifungal agents have been shown to be consistently efficacious as sole or adjuvant topical therapy?

161 i.
- Onychorrhexis: brittle, splitting, or fragmenting claw along the long axis of the claw.
- Onychodystrophy: malformed claw.
- Onycholysis: claw separating from the underlying dermis (corium).
- Onychomadesis: when a claw has sloughed from the digit (P3).
- Onychalgia: pain associated with the claw.
- Paronychia: inflammation of the claw fold and surrounding soft tissue.

ii. Single claw: trauma, infection, foreign body, neoplasia. Multiple claws: genetic, nutritional, autoimmune/immune-mediated disease, endocrine/metabolic, neoplasia.

iii. Since the forelimbs bear more weight than the hindlimbs, a rear digit is preferred for P3 amputation over a forepaw digit. Likewise, any digit other than digit 3 or 4 is recommended as these digits bear more weight than others. Alternatively, if a dewclaw is affected, it should be removed as it bears no weight at all.

iv. An uncommon condition limited to the nails in otherwise healthy dogs with no other skin lesions. It occurs most often in young to middle-aged dogs of all breeds, with German shepherd dogs, rottweilers, schnauzers, and Norwegian Gordon and English setter dogs overrepresented. This dermatopathy is believed to be immune mediated. Initially, 1–2 nails are sloughed (often deemed the result of trauma) with others from multiple paws following suit weeks to months later, resulting in variable lameness. As nails attempt to regrow, they tend to be brittle, frayed, soft, and/or malformed. Secondary bacterial and yeast paronychia accentuates these abnormalities.

162 i. Selection of a systemic antifungal drug and treatment dosing interval. The most commonly used antifungal agents are itraconazole, terbinafine, and fluconazole. Griseofulvin is fungistatic, but its use has become limited due to the availability of drugs that are safer and more effective. It is teratogenic and can be associated with bone marrow suppression. If griseofulvin is used, cats should be tested for FIV and FeLV, which have been associated with a higher risk of bone marrow suppression. Itraconazole is very effective against dermatophytosis. Terbinafine is an allylamine antifungal agent and is also effective against dermatophytes. Fluconazole has efficacy against dermatophytosis; one author has used 10 mg/kg q24h with success. Reported side-effects of azoles and allylamines include occasional vomiting and elevated liver enzymes. Dosing interval is another treatment option that needs to be decided. Both itraconazole and terbinafine have been shown to have residual activity in the skin; treatment has been successful with daily administration until the pet is cured or when used in a pulse therapy format (week on/week off). The major advantage of pulse therapy is client compliance and the clinical observation that cats may have less anorexia and gastrointestinal upset.

ii. *In-vitro* and *in-vivo* studies have regularly shown that enilconazole, lime sulfur, and miconazole-based products are consistently antifungal.

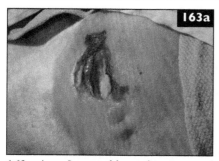

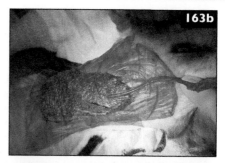

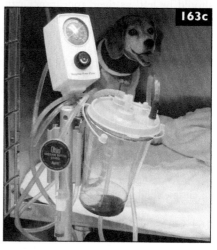

163 An 8-year-old male neutered beagle dog presented on emergency for evaluation of a ventral cervical wound of unknown duration. The dog had been lost for several days prior to presentation. Initial emergency stabilization and triage were performed, and the dog was hemodynamically stable. Radiographs of the cervical region and thoracic cavity were unremarkable other than free gas along the fascial planes of the cervical region. The patient was sedated and the wound examined (**163a**). The head is to the right of the image.

i. Describe the wound based on the wound classification system.

ii. How would you manage this wound?

iii. Initial wound triage was performed and this device was placed onto the wound (**163b, c**). What is this device, and what are the mechanisms of action and recommended settings?

164 A dog weighing 32 kg presents severely depressed, inappetent and with severely crusted skin lesions. You diagnose PF and the only injectable steroid available in your clinic is dexamethasone. What is the equivalent calculated dose of dexamethasone compared with 'immunosuppressive prednisone'? Based on this duration of action, when is the soonest you can start prednisone therapy?

163 i. A class III, contaminated or dirty wound. Wound classification is based on level of contamination and exposure time. Class I is a clean wound or <6 hours duration; class II has significant contamination, or 6–12 hours duration; class III contains gross contamination or >12 hours duration. Critical level of contamination for infected wounds is >10^5 organisms/gram of tissue.

ii. Assess the patient to confirm hemodynamic stability. Thorough physical and directed (orthopedic, neurologic) examinations should be performed prior to sedation. The fur surrounding the wound should be widely clipped; sterile lubricant can be placed in the wound to prevent fur adherence. Debridement of devitalized tissue should be performed using sharp dissection; questionable areas should be left, as their appearance can appear worse initially due to vasospasm and hemodynamic compromise. The wound should be thoroughly lavaged using copious amounts of isotonic solution (lactated Ringer's solution) under moderate pressure. Ideal pressure is 8 psi, which can be generated using a needle (18–20 guage) connected to an intravenous fluid line and pressure bag inflated to 300 mmHg. Submit wound tissue or swab for aerobic and anaerobic bacterial culture and susceptibility analysis. Cover the wound with a sterile dressing and debridement bandage.

iii. A vacuum-assisted closure device, which produces a negative-pressure wound environment with the goals of removing wound fluid, improving tissue circulation, enhancing granulation tissue formation, and increasing bacterial clearance. The system consists of sterile open-cell foam, egress suction tubing, and an occlusive adhesive covering, connected to a suction device. Intermittent suction is recommended at -125 mmHg with a 5 minute ON, 2 minute OFF cycle.

164 Care must be taken when consulting textbooks regarding conversion. It is common for textbooks and on-line sources to list the 'relative anti-inflammatory potency' and the 'equivalent dose'. The relative anti-inflammatory potency of prednisone is 4 compared with 20–30 for dexamethasone. It is common to use on-line calculators to make conversions and, given this range of 20–30, the equivalent dose can vary. The most common equivalent dose (mg) for dexamethasone is 0.75 for 5 mg prednisone. So the dog's total dose of prednisone is 128 mg (4 mg/kg x 32 kg) or 24 mg of dexamethasone (0.75 mg x 32 kg). Dexamethasone has a long duration of action, with a half-life of >48 hours. Theoretically, prednisone therapy can start in 48 hours.

165 With regard to case **163**, what other options exist for the management of contaminated wounds?

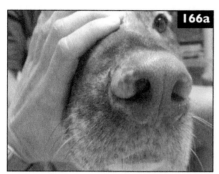 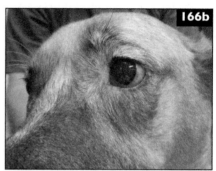

166 A 3-year-old male castrated Rottweiler-cross dog presented for depigmentation of the nasal planum, muzzle (**166a**), hair around the eyes (**166b**), and nails on all four paws. According to the owner, the depigmentation was gradually occurring over the last several months. None of the lesion sites were noted to be pruritic or painful. The nails were firmly attached at the claw fold; however, the nails had lost their normal black pigment. On examination, the nasal planum maintained its normal cobblestone appearance, but it had changed to a mottled gray-pink color (the owner reported the nose was black). Several white hairs were noted in the periocular areas as well as the muzzle. The remainder of the dog's coat was normal.
i. Based on the clinical appearance, what is the most likely diagnosis?
ii. How is this diagnosis confirmed? What are the defining features?
iii. In what breeds of dogs is this condition common?
iv. What is the treatment for the condition?

165 (1) Local antiseptics such as dilute chlorhexidine (0.005%) have excellent immediate and persistent antimicrobial activity with limited toxicity at dilute concentrations. (2) Tris-EDTA alone or in combination with antimicrobials such as aminoglycosides allows for high local concentrations with limited systemic absorption. Tris-EDTA causes disruption of bacterial cell walls and enhances activity of topical antimicrobials. (3) Sugar/honey's proposed mechanisms include decreasing inflammatory edema, attracting tissue macrophages to cleanse the wound, provision of local energy source, and antibacterial properties related to the liberation of hydrogen peroxide. (4) The proposed physiologic effects of hyperbaric O_2 include enhanced or improved oxygen delivery to cells, antimicrobial effects, stimulation of phagocytosis, stimulation of fibroblasts, modulation of neutrophils, and angiogenesis. (5) Silver's proposed mechanisms of action include potent antimicrobial properties of silver ion, anti-inflammatory biochemical properties (decrease matrix metalloproteinase activity), and increasing wound calcium (increases epithelialization).

166 i. Idiopathic vitiligo; focal depigmentation and concurrent leukotrichia are highly characteristic.
ii. Diagnosis is based on clinical appearance and biopsy confirmation. Histopathology typically shows a marked reduction or complete absence of epidermal melanocytes and melanin. Often, melanin can be seen as fine granular particles in the superficial dermis or, more often, engulfed in the small to moderate numbers of dermal melanophages seen in the biopsy specimen.
iii. The disease is uncommon, but it has been reported in Belgian Tervuren, Rottweiler, German shepherd, and Doberman pinscher dogs. In cats, the condition is rare and most commonly reported in Siamese cats.
iv. There is no treatment; it is a cosmetic condition. Affected animals should be protected from excessive sun exposure. Infant-safe sunscreen can be applied to the affected skin to prevent secondary burn injury and actinic changes. Because of the cosmetic issues, this disease has a much greater impact on the quality of life in people; treatment consists of minimizing lesions and repigmentation of the skin. For people options include medical (topical corticosteroids, systemic steroids, or other immunomodulatory medications, phototherapy, photochemotherapy, laser therapy) and surgical treatments (skin grafting, melanocyte suspension transplantation). Other alternative options include make-up to camouflage the area, psychotherapy for emotional issues associated with this disease, depigmentation (skin lightening) to allow for a more generally cosmetic appearance, and alternative therapies such as herbal/Chinese supplements.

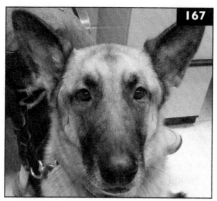

167 A 3-year-old male castrated German shepherd dog is presented for management of year-round chronic otic pruritus (**167**). You perform ear swab cytology today and only shed keratinocytes and a mild amount of ceruminous debris are noted. Otoscopic examination reveals external ear canals of approximately normal diameter with moderately erythematous canal walls and medial pinnae. Both tympanic membranes are intact. The pruritus is only partially responsive to antimicrobial therapy. Regarding the ears, previous treatment of overt infections is helpful and clinical signs recur shortly after therapy has been discontinued.
i. What is the most likely underlying trigger? What other diagnostics would you consider for this patient?
ii. What are your recommendations to control the otic pruritus?

168 A 12-year-old male intact Labrador retriever dog is presented with a 14-day history of acute, non-progressive head tilt. The dog is a working dog, lives largely outside, and is used for hunting, but has not been hunting in the last 3 months. On presentation the dog is bright and interactive and has a normal physical examination except for mild black debris in the external ear canal on both sides. Neurologic examination is normal except for a left head tilt, severe vestibular ataxia with falling to the left, and a rotary nystagmus. The owner has not treated the dog since the onset of the clinical signs and is unaware of any trauma.
i. Based on the findings listed, what is the lesion localization?
ii. What are your top seven differential diagnoses for this patient?

167 i. An allergy. Identification of the underlying allergy is indicated. Two probable causes are food allergy or environmental allergies. A diet trial (novel protein/carbohydrate commercial product, hydrolyzed diet, home-cooked novel protein diet) for at least 6–8 weeks is indicated. If the results of dietary manipulation and subsequent challenge do not provide appreciable benefit, work-up for environmental allergies should be discussed with the owner. Immunotherapy may be a beneficial consideration for the dog given his young age. If the pruritus is localized to the ears, immunotherapy (year-round) should be discussed from a cost-to-benefit standpoint compared with medications that may be needed only intermittently and may be restricted to topical products.
ii. Symptomatic treatment until the cause of the allergic otitis can be identified. This may include antiseptic cleaners and an otic medication containing glucocorticoids. Topical tacrolimus treatment was evaluated in atopic and non-atopic beagle dogs in one study and found to be well tolerated with minimal side-effects.

168 i. This patient is exhibiting signs of vestibular dysfunction. The vestibular system has three main components: vestibular nerve, vestibular nucleus (in the rostral medulla oblongata), and cerebellum (flocculonodular lobe). Lesions are classified as peripheral (involve the receptors or the vestibular nerve) or central (involve the medulla or cerebellum). Central lesions can be subdivided into medulla or cerebellar localization. There are three hallmark signs of medulla localization in veterinary species: paresis, proprioceptive deficits, and mentation changes. Diseases affecting the cerebellum may also show proprioceptive deficits, but hypermetria and intention tremors are often also present. Paresis and proprioceptive deficits occur because of disruption of the descending upper motor neuron or ascending sensory tracts, respectively, coursing through the brainstem. These tracts are paired; therefore, if an animal has a left head tilt, a left hemiparesis and/or left side proprioceptive deficit would be expected. Mentation changes occur with damage to the reticular activating system, which maintains the level of consciousness; therefore, damage can result in the animal being obtunded, stuporous, or comatose. Patients with central disease can have one or more of these findings; however, if any of these findings are present, central localization should be assumed. The direction or phase of nystagmus or the presence of other cranial nerve deficits is not a consideration when localizing a lesion. This dog has a normal neurologic examination except for a left head tilt, nystagmus, and ataxia, which indicates a left peripheral vestibular lesion.
ii. Otitis interna, trauma, foreign body, hypothyroidism, neuritis (immune mediated versus infectious), neoplasia (e.g. lymphoma, nerve sheath tumor), and, less commonly, idiopathic vestibular disease due to the lack of improvement.

169 A 3-year-old male castrated pug-cross dog presented for severe pruritus of 1-year duration. The dog had caused marked self-traumatic lesions including excoriations and erosions over the lateral aspects of both forelimbs from the elbow to the shoulder blades and along the dorsal cervical region. The lesions were hyperpigmented in the center and surrounded by an erythematous border (**169**). The lesions had not responded to appropriate infection control (for both bacterial infection and yeast overgrowth) and effective flea and mite control had ruled out ectoparasite infestation. The

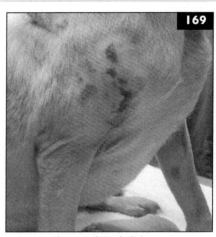

dog had not benefitted from a strict novel protein diet trial and did not improve when corticosteroids were administered, even when administered at high anti-inflammatory/low immunosuppressive doses.

i. Based on the clinical appearance of the lesions, what are proposed differential diagnoses for this patient?

ii. Skin biopsy samples revealed 'epidermal hyperplasia and acanthosis, diffuse, marked, chronic, with hypergranulosis, pigmentation of the basal layers and orthokeratotic hyperkeratosis' consistent with chronic self-trauma. No evidence of vasculitis was detected on multiple biopsy samples. MRI was pursued, which showed Chiari-like malformation and moderate syringomyelia. What are Chiari-like malformation and syringomyelia?

iii. How does this abnormal finding relate to the cutaneous lesions noted in the patient?

170 Desmosomes are adhesion molecules present in all layers of the epidermis. These structures are responsible for cell-to-cell adhesion of epidermal keratinocytes.

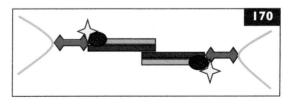

i. What molecules are incorporated into the desmosomal unit (**170**)?

ii. What is the difference between a desmosome, a hemidesmosome, and a corneodesmosome?

Answers: 169, 170

169 i. Vasculitis/vasculopathy, immune-mediate disease (PF, eosinophilic pustulosis, linear acantholytic pustular dermatosis, lupus), allergic skin disease, neuropathy, neoplasia (cutaneous epitheliotropic T-cell lymphoma).

ii. Occipital bone hypoplasia, which results in a portion of the cerebellum descending through the foramen magnum. This malformation results in abnormal CSF flow through the spinal canal. Syringomyelia describes cystic accumulation of fluid or cavitation within the spinal cord.

iii. There are several classifications of pruritus including neurogenic pruritus, which is caused directly by diseases of central structures in the CNS, and neuropathic pruritus, which is caused by damage to the afferent fibers of the peripheral nerves or spinal cord, which transmit pruritus to the skin. Although the exact pathogenesis of pruritus due to Chiari-like malformation and syringomyelia remains unclear, it is suspected that the malformation leads to damage of the dorsal horn and crossing of the spinothalamic fibers, and results in interference of processing of sensory information to and from the skin. This interference causes paraesthesia and resultant scratching. Whether the scratching is due to pain or pruritus is unclear, as these two sensations are very closely related. Cervical/cranial hyperesthesia is seen in approximately 86% of dogs with Chiari-like malformation and syringomyelia, whereas scratching is seen in approximately 62%.

170 i. The desmosomal unit is composed of two compartments: the intracellular plaque and the extracellular core. Plakoglobin and plakophilin bind to intermediate filaments in the intracellular portion of the cell and then bind on the opposite side to desmoplakin. These structures make up the inner dense plaque of the desmosome. Desmoplakin binds to desmocollin and desmoglein, which also bind to each other, to span the extracellular space, forming the core of the desmosome. Different forms of the various molecules are expressed in different layers of the epidermis. Basal cells primarily express desmoglein 2 and 3 and desmocollin II. Cells in the spinous layer express both desmoglein 1 and 3 and desmocollins I, II, and III. In more superficial layers of the epidermis, desmoglein 1 is expressed in greater abundance compared with desmoglein 3. Desmoplakin I and II molecules are expressed in all layers of the epidermis.

ii. A desmosome is responsible for anchoring two neighboring keratinocytes together. They are present in all layers of the epidermis, but are most prominent in the stratum spinosum (desmosomes give this layer its characteristic 'spiny' appearance). A hemidesmosome anchors basal keratinocytes to the basement membrane. They provide a structural link between the extracellular matrix molecules (plectin, integrin, bullous pemphigoid antigens) and keratin intermediate filaments. Corneodesmosomes are modified versions of normal desmosomes and are important for maintaining effective and appropriate desquamation of the stratum corneum cells.

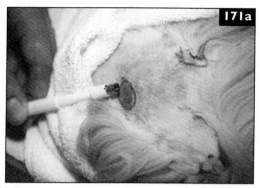

171 A 4-year-old Persian cat was presented for the problem of acute onset of fever, lethargy, and anorexia of 2 days' duration. At the time of examination, the skin was markedly erythematous, painful with even minimal manipulation, and easily torn. During the examination the cat struggled; the skin on the dorsal, neck avulsed from the neck to the dorsal thoracolumbar area. A positive Nikolsky's sign was elicited. Prior to this episode the only abnormality was an eosinophilic granuloma on the lip. The lesion had been only minimally responsive to previously administered glucocorticoids. Prior to referral a diet change had occurred and the cat developed diarrhea, presumably from the diet change. Tylosin powder had been administered to control the diarrhea. A 6-mm skin biopsy was obtained; the biopsy site expanded to 25 mm after sampling due to the extreme fragility of the skin (171a).
i. What are the differential diagnoses for the skin disease?
ii. What is a Nikolsky's sign?
iii. The histologic description of the skin biopsy showed hydropic degeneration of basal epidermal cells, full-thickness coagulation necrosis of the epidermis, minimal inflammation, and separation of the dermal–epidermal junction. What is the diagnosis, and how is this disease managed? What is the prognosis?

172 Desmosomes have important implications in certain dermatologic diseases. In which diseases of dogs and cats do desmosome functions (or dysfunction) contribute to the pathogenesis? What is the pathogenesis of these conditions as it relates to desmosome molecules?

171 i. Inherited collagen defect (i.e. EDS), idiopathic skin fragility syndrome, hyperadrenocorticism. This case is complicated by the fact that the cat shows signs of systemic illness; the differential diagnosis list should be expanded to include drug eruption, TEN, and EM.

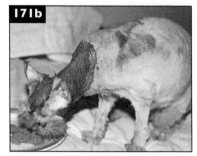

ii. Nikolsky's sign is elicited by applying pressure to the edge of a vesicle, bulla, or patch of skin. It is positive when the outer layer of the skin is easily rubbed off or pushed away. A positive 'Nikolsky's sign' indicates poor cell cohesion; it is often seen in pemphigus, TEN, EM, or drug reactions.

iii. TEN. Wound management and supportive care are necessary. The prognosis is considered poor to guarded. In this case, TEN was presumed due to tylosin administration. Because of the extreme fragility of the skin, a large defect was created when the hair coat was clipped (**171b**). To prevent further tearing of the skin, sterile wound bandages were applied and secured with surgical stockinet material. Withdrawal of tylosin resulted in return of the cat's appetite within 24 hours. Silver sulfadiazine was used to control wound infection. Over the next 6 months the cat's wounds contracted; the only defect post resolution was contraction of the skin between the ears.

172 The most common diseases are the pemphigus complex of diseases (PF, pemphigus vulgaris, paraneoplastic pemphigus). The acantholytic feature of these diseases is due to targeted autoantibodies against various components of the desmosome molecules, leading to detachment of the desmosomes and separation of keratinocytes from neighboring cells. For pemphigus vulgaris, desmoglein 3 has been identified as the major autoantigen in dogs as well as in people. The same molecule has also been implicated as one of the autoantigens in paraneoplastic pemphigus along with other plakins including envoplakin and periplakin. In people, desmoglein 1 is the major autoantigen in PF. Recently, desmocollin I has been identified as one of the major autoantigens in PF in the dog. Darier's disease is a rare genodermatosis that has been reported in both people and dogs. The condition presents as hyperplastic skin with crusted and scaly plaques. Desmosomes are rare or absent; cleft formation and detachment of keratinocytes occur in multiple layers of the epidermis. *Trichophyton* spp. dermatophytes and *Staphylococcus pseudintermedius* bacterial organisms each produce proteolytic enzymes that can disrupt the adhesive properties of desmosomes. This is seen in superficial pustular dermatophytosis and bullous impetigo exfoliative pyoderma; both conditions have been reported in dogs.

173 A 5-year-old male Yorkshire terrier dog presented for depression, lethargy, anorexia, and lameness of 5 days' duration. Prior to presentation, the dog was healthy and had no previous medical problems. Physical examination revealed an elevated rectal temperature, petechial and ecchymotic hemorrhages over the body, peripheral lymphadenopathy, cough, and the facial lesions shown (**173**). Examination of the mouth revealed pale gums, wide-

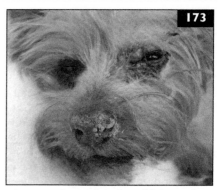

spread petechial hemorrhages, ulcers, erosions, and vesicles. In addition, there were central areas of necrosis and ulceration on the foot pads. The dog was not receiving any medications and flea and tick control consisted of manual removal of fleas and ticks by the owner.

i. What are the most common viral tick-borne pathogens and their current geographic distributions?

ii. What are the most common bacterial tick-borne pathogens and their current common geographic distributions?

iii. What are the most common protozoan tick-borne pathogens and their current geographic distribution?

iv. What is a 'dry ice tick trap' and a 'tick drag'?

174 An IDT is performed on a 3-year-old male castrated Labrador retriever dog with a history and clinical signs consistent with AD. Twenty-five minutes after the test is complete the dog has very strong positive reactions to house dust mites (*D. farinae*) and storage mites (*Acarus* and *Lepidoglyphus* spp.). At the time of discharge, the dog does not have any erythema or lingering wheal formation from the IDT. Approximately 6 hours after discharge, the owner calls and reports that at the site of the IDT there are multiple focal areas of erythema and swelling; the dog is intensely pruritic.

i. How do you explain to the owner what has happened?

ii. What is the typical approach to treatment? How do you manage this?

173 i. Tick-borne encephalitis (central Europe), louping ill virus (GB, Ireland).
ii. *Borrelia* spp. (USA, Europe, Asia, Japan, Canada, Africa, Brazil), *Anaplasma* spp. (USA, Europe, South America, Africa, Middle East, Southeast Asia), *Rickettsia* spp. (USA, Latin America, Central and South America, Europe, Africa, India, parts of South East Asia).
iii. *Babesia* spp. (Europe, tropical and subtropical regions, USA, parts of Africa, Japan), *Hepatozoon* spp. (southern Europe, Japan, Thailand, Philippines, India, Africa, Middle East, South America, southern USA).
iv. Both are used to decrease the population of ticks in a small area without using pesticides. A dry ice tick trap is one of many non-pesticide methods for local control of ticks in the environment and it takes advantage of the tick's natural attraction to carbon dioxide. The edge of a square wooden board is covered with strips of masking tape or duck tape sticky side up. One kilogram of dry ice is placed in a plastic bucket with 10–20 holes punched near the bottom. The bucket is placed on the board and ticks are trapped in the sticky tape. The trap will last for approximately 2–3 hours. For a tick drag, light colored flannel cloth is dragged across vegetation where ticks may be waiting for a host. The ticks will attach themselves to the cloth. After 'dragging the area', the cloth can be burned or sprayed with an insecticide.

174 i. This dog is experiencing a late-phase reaction to the allergens injected during the IDT. This late-phase reaction is IgE mediated and is thought to be caused by mast cell degranulation, chemoattraction, and inflammatory cell infiltration. In human studies it has been shown that the incidence of late-phase reaction increases with increasing concentration of injected allergen. In people, if an individual has a late-phase reaction, it is believed to be associated with a higher degree of allergen hypersensitivity. One study showed that 40% of atopic dogs had late-phase reactions after intradermal injection of house dust mite allergen.
ii. It is important to prevent self-trauma to the affected area from biting, licking, chewing, and scratching, so an Elizabethan collar or shirt may be used. If the clinical signs are mild, cold compressing may provide some temporary relief. Topical corticosteroids (sprays, gels, lotions) may help ease the erythema and pruritus. If that does not provide relief, a short course of an anti-inflammatory dose of oral corticosteroids (prednisone or prednisolone) can be considered. The authors routinely ask owners to take digital pictures if any late-phase reactions are seen after discharge. The late-phase reaction provides additional information about the IDT and can help with the formulation of immunotherapy.

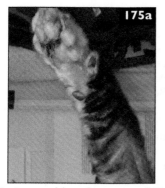
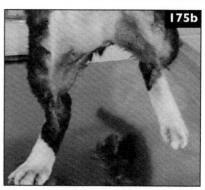

175 A 6-year-old male castrated Devon Rex cat presents for persistent waxy debris on the skin and overgrooming of all four limbs (175a, b). Skin cytology is performed and numerous yeast organisms are noted from around the nail folds. Although the owners have not reported overt signs of otitis externa, you notice on physical examination that both external ear canals contain a large amount of dark brown, waxy debris. Similar organisms are noted on ear swab cytology.
i. What breeds of cats are noted for *Malassezia* overgrowth of the skin and ear canals?
ii. What species of *Malassezia* have been reported in cats?
iii. How is the disease condition managed typically?

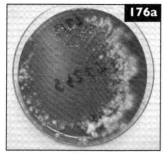
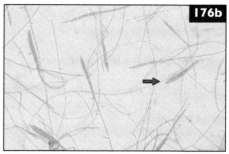

176 This fungal culture plate (176a) was inoculated 18 days ago from a cat undergoing both systemic and topical treatment for dermatophytosis. Note the lack of growth in the center and the ring of fungal growth on the margins of the plate. Cytologic examination of the growth is shown (176b). The growth on this plate was subcultured onto Sabouraud's dextrose agar, incubated at 37°C, and confirmed to be *M. canis*. What was happening with the treatment culture?

183

175 i. Although any cat with signs of otitis externa may have overgrowth of *Malassezia* on cytology, certain breeds tend to be more prone to this superficial mycosis. Devon Rex cats and Sphynx cats have a higher likelihood of *Malassezia* overgrowth when compared with other domestic cat breeds. When similar breeds are assessed (e.g. Devon versus Cornish Rex cats), the Devon Rex still shows higher prevalence of *Malassezia* overgrowth. Both Devon Rex and Sphynx cats are prone to primary cornification defects (primary seborrhea), which likely accounts for concurrent *Malassezia* overgrowth; more cutaneous nutrients serve as an ideal environment for microbial overgrowth. Although earlier reports implied that concurrent disease states (e.g. diabetes mellitus, hyperthyroidism) increased the likelihood of *Malassezia* overgrowth, a more recent study could not substantiate this claim. This study did, however, corroborate the association of feline paraneoplastic alopecia and cutaneous *Malassezia* overgrowth irrespective of breed.

ii. *M. pachydermatis, M. sympodialis, M. globosa, M. furfur, M. nana, M. slooffiae, M. obtusa*, and *M. restricta*.

iii. Although topical therapy with antifungal rinses and anti-seborrheic agents can be beneficial, this is difficult in many cats, making treatment less effective. Itraconazole administration has been effective; response to therapy supports a diagnosis of *Malassezia* overgrowth in these cats in a similar fashion to the response to treatment of the disease in dogs. Other azole derivatives or terbinafine may also be effective.

176 This is a very common finding in toothbrush cultures obtained from animals receiving topical therapy. First, growth of the dermatophyte is often delayed because of treatment. Second, both gross and microscopic growth are altered in appearance. In this case, the plates were inoculated from the center outwards towards the margins of the plate. Growth was inhibited in the center of the plate due to trace amounts of topical antifungal solution alone or on infective spores being deposited onto the plate. As the inoculation moved to the margins of the plate, trace solution and/or infective spores not covered in antifungal solution were deposited on the plate and allowed to grow. Lack of sporulation is a common finding in animals undergoing treatment, especially in the later stages of therapy. The arrow is identifying the swollen end of a hypha where a dermatophyte macroconidium is trying to develop. This thickened 'finger-like' projection is typical of *M. canis* colonies incubated at suboptimal temperatures or exposed to antifungal therapies.

177 The tail of an atopic golden retriever dog is shown (177). What is unusual about the tail, and what do you suspect is the cause?

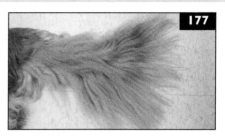

178 A 6-year-old male castrated American bulldog was presented for a 6-month history of progressive nodular skin disease (178a, b). The owner reported that nodules initially presented over the limbs and head but have spread to involve most body regions. Lesions begin as firm nodules that enlarge, ulcerate, and become exudative and matted with a thick adherent crust. Multiple courses of systemic antibiotics had not been beneficial. Although oral corticosteroids (anti-inflammatory dose) seemed to result in a slight reduction in lesion size, the nodules never completely regressed. The dog had a history of traveling out of the local region prior to lesion development; however, other household dogs had not

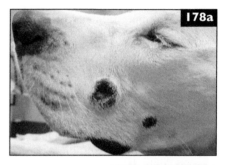

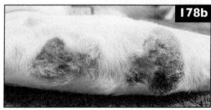

been similarly affected. More recently, the dog had developed clinical signs of systemic illness including gastrointestinal upset and decreased activity. Pruritus was not a reported feature; however, the owner felt the dog was painful where nodules were present.
i. What are your differential diagnoses for this patient?
ii. What diagnostic testing would you recommend?
iii. Skin biopsy of the nodules showed sheets of neoplastic round cells with diffuse and perivascular distribution. Occasional small aggregates of neoplastic cells were found within the epidermis. The cells had large round to oval nuclei with multiple large nucleoli and a moderate amount of pale cytoplasm. Mitotic index was high. The cells infiltrated into follicular, apocrine gland, and sebaceous epithelium. Immunohistochemical staining was positive for CD3 in the neoplastic cells. Given this report, what is the diagnosis?
iv. What treatment options are available for this condition, and what is the prognosis?

177 It is exhibiting hypertrichosis. The most common cause of hypertrichosis in dogs is cyclosporine administration. At the time of presentation, the dog had been receiving 5 mg/kg cyclosporine q24h for 2 years for management of AD. If this is the only clinical abnormality noted, likely no change in therapy is necessary.

178 i. Infectious (deep fungal including blastomycosis, cryptococcosis, histoplasmosis, coccidioidomycosis; opportunistic fungal, eumycotic mycetoma, dermatophytic pseudomycetoma; atypical bacteria including botryomycosis, mycobacterial infection, nocardiosis, actinomycosis, canine leproid granuloma, L-form infection); inflammatory (cutaneous histiocytosis, sterile pyogranuloma/granuloma syndrome); neoplasia (cutaneous epitheliotropic T-cell lymphoma, MCT).
ii. Cytologic impression and FNA, routine aerobic bacterial cultures, and cultures for atypical bacterial infections. Laboratory personnel should be alerted to the possible contagious nature of the organism (particularly for deep fungal mycoses). Skin biopsy is recommended as this will most rapidly differentiate infectious versus neoplastic diseases.
iii. Epitheliotropic T-cell lymphoma.
iv. Various treatment protocols have been tried, but few have reported good efficacy. In general, the prognosis is poor, with mean survival time from diagnosis of months to 2 years. Palliative options include supplementation with high concentrations of linoleic acid or administration of corticosteroids (e.g. prednisone or prednisolone). A recent study demonstrated the presence of retinoid receptors in tumors of dogs diagnosed with cutaneous lymphoma; although not thoroughly investigated, retinoid receptor binding drugs may be beneficial. Lomustine (CCNU) is an alkylating agent that has been one of the more promising treatment options for canine cutaneous lymphoma. Higher dosing protocols have increased efficacy, with a response rate of 78–83% reported. The effect of this treatment on survival has not been reported. Lymphoma in both dogs and people is a highly radiosensitive neoplasia. Newer radiation delivery systems may allow this possibility to be a more favorable option, as treatment can be tailored to the individual patient while minimizing damage to surrounding normal tissues.

179 Owners are often frustrated by cases of generalized demodicosis that 'fail to resolve' with the treatment that has been prescribed. There is a small population of dogs that will have chronic demodicosis (i.e. dogs that apparently cure but continually relapse) due to an impaired skin immune system. Excluding these dogs, when presented with a case of 'refractory demodicosis', what other reasons should be discussed with the owner and investigated?

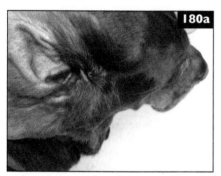 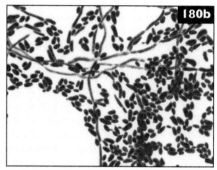

180 A 5-year-old male neutered basset hound dog was presented for the problem of persistent otic pruritus (>1 year) manifested by 'ear flapping' (**180a**). The dog had no other clinical signs of skin disease. Otic examination revealed diffuse erythema from the ear pinnae to the tympanic membrane. Initial otic cytology was unremarkable and did not reveal any inflammatory cells or organisms. The owners had cleaned the dog's ears daily since it was a puppy. The owners declined further diagnostics. Because of the possibility that either the ear cleaning procedure and/or a topical ear cleaner might be causing a local allergic/irritant reaction, all ear cleaning was discontinued for 14 days. Approximately 10 days after the initial visit, the owners presented the dog because of increasing ear pruritus, odor, and marked ceruminous exudate. Ear swab cytology revealed too many to count *Malassezia* organisms. The dog was sedated, the ears cleaned, and a treatment protocol of oral ketoconazole (5 mg/kg q24h for 21 days) and topical ear steroids (dexamethasone and propylene glycol) and topical miconazole solution was prescribed. The dog was re-examined at the end of treatment and the owners reported a marked reduction in ear pruritus, but persistence of a ceruminous exudate. Repeat ear cytology is shown (**180b**). Identify the organisms.

179 Common reasons for treatment 'failure' with generalized demodicosis include:
- Failure to address concurrent bacterial pyoderma. Bacterial pyoderma (superficial or deep) is frequently noted concurrently with generalized demodicosis. If infection is not addressed, *Demodex* mites will persist. It is difficult for treatment to reach therapeutic concentrations in the skin when a large amount of purulent material is also present.
- Failure to prescribe an adequate dose of miticide medication. For example, ivermectin is commonly used for the treatment of demodicosis; however, the dosage needs to be much higher than for other parasitic infestations. Dosage for heartworm prevention is approximately 0.6 mg/kg once every 30 days; for sarcoptic mange it is 0.2–0.3 mg/kg PO or SC once every 7–14 days for 6–8 weeks; for demodicosis it is 0.3–0.6 mg/kg q24h for average treatment duration of 7 months.
- Failure to treat long enough. The goal of treatment is to achieve 2–3 consecutive negative skin scrapings, 2–4 weeks apart. Negative skin scraping means no mites of any life stage present, either alive or dead.
- Failure to identify and address concurrent medical disease. This is particularly true for cases of adult-onset generalized demodicosis.
- Premature discontinuation of treatment by owners. When the dog 'looks better' owners may think treatment can be discontinued. It is important to educate owners from the beginning that their dog will reach a clinical cure much sooner than it will reach a parasitic cure.
- Failure to identify a concurrent disease causing immunosuppression, or concurrent illness being treated with immunosuppressant therapy (e.g. neoplasia).

180 *Candida* in large numbers with smaller numbers of *Malassezia*. *Malasssezia* are bottle-shaped, thick-walled, up to 5 µm in length, and reproduce by monopolar budding on a broad base. *M. pachydermatis* is the only member of the genus that grows on Sabouraud dextrose agar without lipid supplementation. *Candida* pseudohyphae show distinct points of constriction often resembling sausage links. They have narrow base budding, making it easy to distinguish from *Malassezia*. *Candida* blastoconidia, or yeast-like cells, are larger than *Malassezia*. In this case, a culture isolated both *Malassezia* and *Candida* (*C. tropicalis*); susceptibility testing revealed that both organisms were susceptible to all antifungal drugs tested. *Candida* spp. are common commensals of animals, often found at the mucosal junctions. Candidiasis is often observed in immunocompromised individuals. During the work-up of this case it was found that the dog had autoimmune hemolytic anemia.

181 A 5-year-old male neutered Labrador retriever dog with an incompletely excised grade II mast cell tumor of the distal limb was presented for consultation. The owners were considering definitive radiation therapy treatment (attempt to sterilize the tumor field, with the goal of curing residual microscopic neoplasia, with typical treatment dose amounts exceeding 45 Gy within 3–4 weeks) and wanted an insight into the cutaneous toxicity associated with treatment.
i. What is the normal progression of acute radiation-induced skin reactions?
ii. What is the basic pathobiology of radiation-induced injury to the skin?

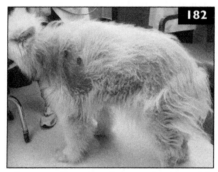

182 A 6-year-old female spayed samoyed dog presents with a progressive history of non-pruritic skin and 'hair that has been falling out, often in clumps'. No other signs of systemic illness are reported. On physical examination there is partial to complete alopecia primarily affecting the truncal region (**182**). All of the head and all four limbs have been spared. The skin underlying alopecia appears normal with no evidence of inflammatory changes. The hair coat is sparse; what hair remains has a 'wooly' appearance. Skin scrapings are negative on multiple sites sampled. Surface skin cytology does not reveal any infection or microbial overgrowth.
i. Multiple skin biopsy specimens are obtained from normal and affected areas. The affected regions show epidermis of a normal thickness with moderate hyperpigmentation. Most of the hair follicles are in haired telogen; however, many show an excess amount of trichilemmal keratinization that is consistent with 'flame follicle' appearance. Based on this description, what is the diagnosis for this patient?
ii. What is the current proposed pathogenesis of this disease in dogs?
iii. What options are there for managing the condition?

181 i. Erythema, dry desquamation, hyper-pigmentation, moist desquamation, skin necrosis (**181**).

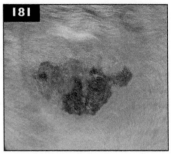

ii. Hierarchical organization exists within the germinal components of the basal and suprabasal layers of the epithelia. A single stem cell in the basal layer of the epidermis is surrounded by a column of daughter or transient amplifying cells (progenitor cells), which continue through the maturation/cornification process. The radiosensitivity of cells in these layers decreases during the maturation process, leaving them less prone to injury and toxicity effects; cells at most risk are those in the germinal (basal) layer or stem cells. The preferential depletion of cells in the stem cell and early progenitor cell compartments results in a progressive decline in the number of cells available for terminal differentiation (fewer cells becoming fully cornified keratinocytes). This can eventually have a negative impact on the protective barrier function of the skin, leaving the patient at risk for secondary complications (e.g. infections, dehydration, solar injury). Barrier function is maintained until post-mitotic cells are lost through continuing normal cell turnover.

182 i. Alopecia X (or hair cycle arrest).
ii. The exact pathogenesis is not known. The disease presents with bilaterally symmetrical, non-inflammatory hair loss resembling the appearance of 'endocrine alopecia', in which the head and limbs are spared. There appears to be a genetic influence, as this disease is seen almost exclusively in Nordic dog breeds with plush double coats (samoyed, pomeranian, keeshond); familial association has also been documented. Several studies have failed to identify the causative gene. Estrogen receptor presence does not appear to be associated with the disease and antagonism of the receptors does not appear to influence hair regrowth. Based on response to treatment trials, there is suspicion that abnormal adrenal function may be involved; however, this has not been well documented.
iii. In some dogs where adrenal hormone abnormalities have been documented, treatment with either mitotane or trilostane has resulted in hair regrowth. Treatment risks include development of hypoadrenocorticism and/or adrenal necrosis. Monitoring is necessary to evaluate treatment efficacy and adverse reactions. In patients without any evidence of systemic illness and no other abnormalities other than hair loss, it is questionable whether this aggressive treatment is necessary. Many clinicians consider alopecia X (different from atypical hyperadrenocorticism) a cosmetic disease. Melatonin supplementation (3–6 mg/dog q12–24h) has been beneficial in some patients; side-effects may include sedation. 'Sweater therapy' has been helpful for some dogs and their owners.

183 i. What determines the severity of radiation-induced injury (see also case **181**)?
ii. What determines the rate at which acute injury occurs?

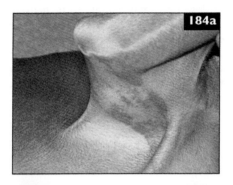

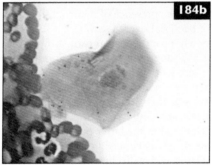

184 The axillary area of a 6-year-old female spayed mixed-breed dog is shown (**184a**). The dog lives indoors. The lesions shown develop in late August through October and are pruritic. The owners report only mild facial and otic pruritus, but are most concerned about the recurrent axillary lesions. The clinical signs began when the dog was 1 year of age and consistently resolve once the weather becomes cold. In the past, the clinical signs have been well managed by systemic glucocorticoids, but the owners are reluctant to administer them due to annoying side-effects (polyuria, polydipsia). The dog receives year-round flea and tick control and skin scrapings are negative. Skin cytology from an impression smear is shown (**184b**).
i. What is the interpretation of the skin cytology?
ii. What is the cause of the dog's recurrent skin lesions?
iii. What are important points to discuss with the client regarding specialized diagnostic testing?

183 i. The severity depends both on the extent of stem and progenitor cell depletion (how many cells are lost from the germinal layer and do not mature/complete the cornification process) and the length of delay of maturation from stem cell to fully differentiated keratinocyte. Severity of injury increases with dose (how much total radiation is delivered to the site, measured in Gy), but dose fractionation (breaking up the total dose into smaller units to be delivered over an extended time period) can decrease the adverse effects by allowing regeneration of the stem cell and progenitor cell compartments over the course of radiotherapy. In essence, this allows for the skin to recover. Dose fraction schedules are considerably more coarse (larger units of radiation delivered in fewer treatment sessions) in veterinary medicine compared with our human counterparts (smaller units delivered more frequently).

ii. It is predominantly independent of dose and more determined by loss of cells from the terminally differentiated compartment. The more cells that are destroyed from the germinal cell layers, the higher is the likelihood that radiation-induced skin injury will occur. This can happen both with comparatively low radiation delivery doses (e.g. 15 Gy) as well as with high (e.g. 45Gy) doses.

184 i. Bacterial pyoderma. The presence of neutrophils is compelling evidence that the cocci are more than bacterial overgrowth.

ii. Seasonal AD. The newly proposed diagnostic criteria for AD include: onset of signs under 3 years of age; dog living mostly indoors; glucocorticoid-responsive pruritus; pruritus that precedes development of lesions; affected front feet; affected ear pinnae; non-affected ear margins; non-affected dorsolumbar area. In a dog with recurrent seasonal pruritus occurring in the fall (autumn), the two most common differential diagnoses would be seasonal AD and fleas. Administration of year-round flea prevention makes the latter possibility less likely.

iii. In general, diagnosis of AD is clinical; allergy testing is performed to identify allergens for ASIT. Testing is usually limited to 50–60 allergens. Removal of a weed or tree from the dog's immediate home will not prevent exposure to the allergen. Pollen particles are airborne and can travel hundreds of miles. Reasons for ASIT in dogs with seasonal atopy include: clinical signs cannot be managed medically; failure to respond to therapy regardless of the severity of the pruritus; therapy is contraindicated (e.g. diabetic dog and steroids); effective therapy alters performance or behavior (e.g. steroid aggression, antihistamines, sleepiness or hyperactivity). Other key points to stress are that ASIT is year-round and currently presumed to be lifelong therapy; it can take 3–12 months to see maximum benefit.

185 A 7-year-old female spayed mixed-breed boxer dog presents for crusting skin lesions and ear margins that bleed easily during normal activity. The dog had been acquired from a rescue organization several months prior to presentation, therefore her previous history is unknown. At the time of adoption, the dog was diagnosed with heartworm disease and numerous microfilaria were noted on a blood smear. The dog has since been treated for the microfilariasis and appears to be in good overall health. On physical examination, both pinnae are noted to be crusted and scalloped along with margins (185a); the ear tips bleed with minimal manipulation. The tip of the nose is irregular, with erosions and loss of normal cobblestone architecture (185b). The tip of the tail is also crusted and alopecic. There is a near complete absence of claws on all digits of all four paws (185c). Based on the distribution of skin lesions, you make a clinical diagnosis of vasculitis/vasculopathy.

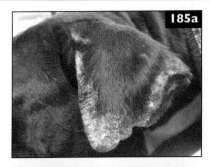

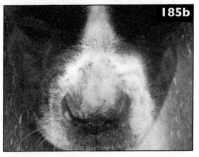

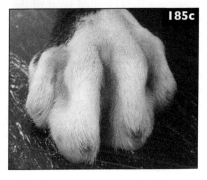

i. There are a number of causes of vasculitis/vasculopathy in the dog. List several infectious etiologies that can cause vasculitis.
ii. List several non-infectious etiologies for vasculitis.
iii. How might you manage the clinical signs in this dog?

186 The process of skin formation involves a series of highly regulated events in order to form a functional epidermal barrier. Defects or abnormalities in the process cause decreased barrier function and can contribute to several dermatologic disease states.
i. Name the four layers of the epidermis.
ii. How do 'keratinization' and 'cornification' differ?
iii. Describe the cellular events involved in cornification.

185 i. Septic vasculitis: deep bacterial pyoderma, Rocky Mountain spotted fever, ehrlichiosis, and *Erysipelothrix rhusiopathiae* in dogs. Neutrophilic immunologic vasculitis is considered to be a non-infectious cause of vasculitis in dogs; however, the condition may be precipitated by viral diseases or leishmaniasis. Vasculopathy of greyhound dogs ('Alabama rot') is due to a shiga-like toxin produced by *Escherichia coli* O157:H7 found in raw diets fed to racing greyhounds. Vasculitis has also been reported in a dog with disseminated histoplasmosis. The severe heartworm disease may also have contributed to the vasculitis/vasculopathy lesions seen in this dog; if thrombi from microfilarial death form, they could potentially become lodged in smaller vessels, leading to development of cutaneous lesions.
ii. SLE, rheumatoid arthritis, paraneoplastic syndromes, cryoglobulinemia/cryofibrinogenemia, drug reactions, ischemic dermatopathy of Jack Russell terrier dogs, dermatomyositis, familial vasculopathy of German shepherd dogs, post-rabies vaccine induced.
iii. Treat infections if identified. Lesions are mild and may be managed with a combination of tetracycline or doxycycline and niacinamide. Pentoxifylline is also an option. If lesions worsen, more aggressive immunosuppressive therapy (prednisone) can be used.

186 i. From deep to superficial: strata basale, spinosum, granulosum, and corneum.
ii. 'Keratinization' is a series of genetically programed events through which keratinocytes in the basal layer of the epidermis differentiate, mature, and die, producing the cornified layer of the epidermis (stratum corneum). 'Cornification' includes keratinization and all of the steps in the formation of the cornified epidermal envelope.
iii. In keratinization, epidermal cells mature from basal cells to flattened, dead corneocytes. During maturation, structural proteins and lipids are expressed. In the basal layer, cells are active with high mitotic ability. On leaving the basal layer, they lose mitotic ability and progress to terminally differentiated corneocytes. In the spinous layer, lamellar granules contain precursors to lipids, proteins, free fatty acids, and enzymes; these contents will form the cornified envelope. In the granular layer, lamellar granules fuse with the cell membrane. Contents are exocytosed and utilized in cornified envelope formation. Keratohyalin granules containing profilaggrin, loricrin, and keratin filaments are formed in this layer and go on to form the cornified envelope. Protein accounts for 90% of the cornified envelope; these covalently cross-linked polymers are insoluble, lending to the protective epidermal barrier. Lipid accounts for the other 10%; extruded contents of lamellar granules (ceramides, free fatty acids, cholesterol) interdigitate with intracellular lipids to adhere the structure to corneocytes and complete the epidermal barrier.

187 A current controversy in the literature is what should be the correct term to describe cats with allergic skin disease caused by something other than fleas or food. Some argue that the term feline 'atopic dermatitis' is inaccurate and a more appropriate term should be used. What are the arguments for and against this controversy?

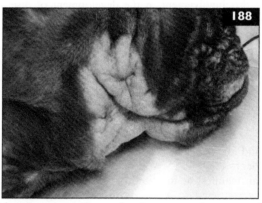

188 A 4-year-old male castrated pug dog is presented to your clinic. The owner reports she came home from work to find the dog's head and neck 'swollen and red' (**188**). The dog is currently not receiving any medication except for routine flea, tick, and heartworm preventives and there have been no recent vaccinations. The dog has access to the inside of the home and, via a dog door, an outside fenced yard. Except for being intensely pruritic, the dog is otherwise healthy. The subcutaneous masses are firm, but pit and blanch with gentle pressure/palpation.
i. What is the most likely diagnosis? What is the prognosis?
ii. How is this condition manifested?
iii. How do you treat this condition?

187 The term 'feline AD' was first introduced into the literature in 1982. It was used to describe a group of pruritic cats in which intradermal testing for environmental allergens was positive and in which other causes of pruritus (external parasites, infections, flea allergy, food allergy) had been ruled out. In essence, the disease was diagnosed as it is in dogs and people: a clinical diagnosis based on exclusion. In dogs, AD is defined as 'a genetically predisposed inflammatory and pruritic allergic skin disease with characteristic clinical features associated with IgE antibodies most commonly directed against environmental allergens'. IgE has been implicated with regard to development of AD and other allergic skin diseases in cats; however, others argue that this involvement in the development of disease has not been firmly established. The heterogeneity of the feline IgE molecule and lack of positive allergy tests in approximately 35% of cats with a clinical diagnosis of AD are cited as reasons why this disease in cats should have a different terminology. Proposed alternative names include 'feline non-flea/non-food allergic dermatitis' and 'feline non-flea/non-food hypersensitivity dermatosis'. Whatever name is eventually deemed the most appropriate, cats with AD appear to respond similarly to dogs with regard to medical management of the disease as well as response to immunotherapy.

188 i. Urticaria and angioedema. Because the lesions are limited to the skin, the prognosis is excellent.
ii. Anaphylaxis can manifest as localized or generalized reactions. Localized anaphylaxis has signs restricted to a specific tissue or organ, usually at epithelial surfaces. Typically, these reactions include pruritus, urticaria, and angioedema. Maculopapular eruptions and erythroderma can also be seen. These lesions are often found on the ventral abdomen since a thick hair coat can hide lesions on the rest of the body. Generalized anaphylaxis is a systemic hypersensitivity reaction resulting in a shock-like state and involving multiple organ systems. Clinical signs can also include vomiting, diarrhea, urination, respiratory distress, tachycardia, and collapse. A generalized anaphylactic reaction can be fatal if rapid treatment is not initiated.
iii. For a local reaction, antihistamines may be all that is necessary. The animal should be washed or bathed if a topical product (shampoo, spray, gel, ointment) is the inciting cause. If urticaria and/or angioedema is present, glucocorticoids are indicated until signs of the reaction subside. For a generalized anaphylactic reaction, any suspect medication or product must be stopped, oxygen (if respiratory signs are evident) and intravenous fluid therapy should be provided, and glucocorticoid and epinephrine therapy initiated. Careful monitoring of heart rate, respiratory rate, blood pressure, temperature, and urinary output may be required for many hours. With successful intense intervention and supportive care, improvement is typically seen within 1–3 hours.

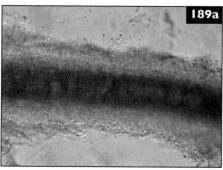

189 These are hairs from a trichogram of a cat (189a). What is the diagnosis?

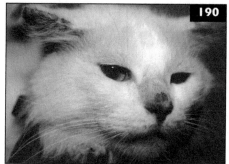

190 A 15-year-old indoor–outdoor cat from a sunny climate has a history of SCC of the ears; 5 years ago the lesions were treated via bilateral partial cosmetic pinnectomy. The cat is now presented for erythematous crusted lesions in the pre-auricular areas and on the nasal planum (190). The cat is receiving year-round flea control. Otic examination of the remaining ear canal is within normal limits. Dermatophyte culture is pending. Impression smears of the lesions are non-diagnostic. Skin biopsy of a lesion from the pre-auricular area reveals findings compatible with actinic dermatitis and from the nose the diagnosis is compatible with SCC.

i. What are the treatment options for feline SCC of the nose, ears, and skin? Which is best?
ii. What is Bowen's disease? What is a key clinical feature?
iii. What is imiquimod?

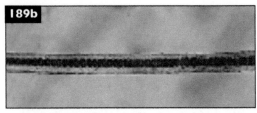

189 Dermatophytosis. Note the large cuff of ectothrix spores surrounding the hair shaft. The margin of the hair shaft is irregular compared with a normal hair (189b).

190 i. Aggressive surgical excision of the affected tissue; this is the best treatment option when available. Surgical removal of nasal lesions is an option depending on the extent of the lesion and whether the lips are involved. Alternative or adjunct therapies include radiation, photodynamic therapy, cryotherapy, and intralesional injection of chemotherapeutic drugs (5-fluorouracil).

ii. Bowen's disease or multicentric SCC *in situ* (MSCCIS) is an uncommon skin disease in cats. It is characterized by multifocal lesions over the head, neck, dorsal thorax, abdomen, and limbs. Lesions are found in haired skin and darkly pigmented skin and are not solar induced. Lesions can be treated with surgical excision. Systemic chemotherapy has shown little benefit. There is some evidence to suggest that bowenoid in situ carcinomas may involve a viral origin.

iii. Imiquimod (an imidazoquinoline amine) is a topical immune modulator that has antiviral and antitumor activity in animals and people. Imiquimod has been used to treat cats with MSCCIS. In one study, 12 cats were treated with 5% imiquimod cream; initial lesions responded in all cats. New lesions developed in 8/12 cats; again lesions responded to imiquimod cream. Adverse effects included local erythema, temporary worsening of lesions, increased liver enzymes, rare neutropenia and vomiting. In a single case report, a cat with both actinic changes and SCC of the pinnae was treated with imiquimod 5% cream; lesions resolved after 12 weeks of therapy. Similar side-effects were seen within the first 3 weeks of therapy. Imiquimod may be an option for therapy for cats with actinic changes, MSCCIS, or SCC when surgery or radiation is not an option.

191 i. What are the most common cutaneous clinical signs associated with feline hyperthyroidism?
ii. How are these clinical signs manifested based on the pathogenesis of hyperthyroidism?

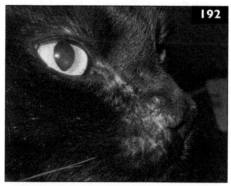

192 A cat was presented for this lesion on its face (**192**). The owner was unable to offer any history. Cytologic findings were non-diagnostic and a skin biopsy specimen was submitted for examination. The microscopic report stated: 'The epidermis is multifocally hyperplastic and ulcerated. Keratinocytes in the epidermis at the margins of the ulcerations are swollen and have enlarged nuclei with pale basophilic glassy intranuclear inclusions and marginating chromatin. The follicular epithelium of hair follicles at sites of ulceration is necrotic, and disassociated aggregates of follicular epithelial cells are brightly eosinophilic and necrotic and adjacent follicular epithelial cells are swollen and have enlarged nuclei with pale basophilic glassy inclusions and marginating chromatin. In the dermis beneath the ulcerations and surrounding necrotic follicles there are scattered mast cells, macrophages, neutrophils, and karyorrhectic debris. Occasional sebaceous glands are also necrotic and nuclei contain viral inclusions'. The morphologic diagnosis was necrotizing and ulcerative dermatitis with intraepithelial intranuclear viral inclusions.
i. What are possible differential diagnoses for the lesions in this cat?
ii. What is the diagnosis based on the macroscopic and microscopic findings?
iii. What other signs might the cat display with this diagnosis?
iv. How might you manage this case?

191 i. Hair coat changes are a common finding in cats with hyperthyroidism. Common clinical signs include patchy alopecia, matted hair, decreased grooming behavior, greasy seborrhea, or a generally unkempt hair coat. Excess dander (**191**) and long, thick claws may also be seen in some cats. Symmetrical non-inflammatory alopecia is not typically associated with hyperthyroidism. Decreased

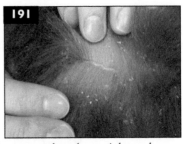

grooming and unkempt coat can possibly lead to secondary bacterial pyoderma, although this is typically less common in cats than dogs. As with other internal diseases, cats with hyperthyroidism may develop outbreaks of *Demodex cati* mites.
ii. Increased protein synthesis and metabolism has been implicated in many clinical symptoms of hyperthyroidism, including cutaneous changes. Epidermal turnover rate can be increased, leading to increased dander, sebaceous gland secretion, and nail growth. In humans, increased vasodilation and generation of heat have also been reported with hyperthyroidism; cats are often noted to have warm skin, particularly in alopecic areas. Changes in internal health, due to any etiology in any species, can affect the cutaneous microflora, leading to other concurrent dermatoses. Bacterial pyoderma and demodicosis are most frequently reported as secondary findings.

192 i. Include infections (e.g. pyoderma, dermatophytosis, dimorphic fungi), cutaneous parasites (e.g. demodicosis), allergic skin disease (flea allergy, cutaneous adverse food reaction, AD), viral-related dermatitis (e.g. herpesvirus), autoimmune dermatoses (e.g. PF), and neoplasia (e.g. SCC, cutaneous lymphoma).
ii. Herpesvirus 1-associated dermatitis (feline rhinotracheitis virus). Intranuclear viral inclusion bodies are seen with herpesvirus. Other viruses affecting the skin of cats, such as pox and papilloma, have intracytoplasmic viral inclusions.
iii. In addition to ulcerative papules on periocular and perinasal skin, cats with Herpesvirus 1-associated dermatitis might present with depression, lethargy, anorexia, fever, conjunctivitis, and repeated sneezing episodes. Keratitis, muco-purulent ocular and nasal discharge, crusting of nares, and oral ulcers may also be seen. Rarely, cutaneous skin ulcers distant from the face and oral cavity may be seen. Affected cats often have a history of upper respiratory disease.
iv. Oral famciclovir (adult cat, 125 mg PO q8–12h; kitten, 25–40 mg/kg PO q8–12h) has shown the most promise for this skin disease. Systemic clindamycin, doxycycline, or amoxicillin–clavulanate may be coadministered with famciclovir for chronic 'snufflers'. Anecdotally, docosanol 10% cream applied topically to early skin lesions may reduce the extent and severity of disease. Topical ophthalmic medication (e.g. lubrication, antibiotics) is used commonly for keratitis and conjunctivitis.

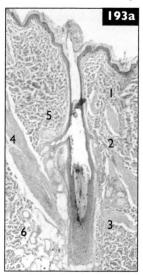 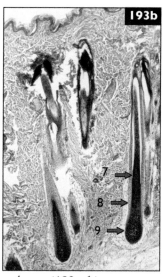

193 Diagrams of a canine hair follicle are shown (**193a, b**).
i. Identify the structures labeled 1–9. Is this a primary or secondary hair?
ii. What are the three tightly regulated phases of hair growth in the dog?
iii. On a skin biopsy report, luminal folliculitis is described. What structures are involved in luminal folliculitis, and what are your differential diagnoses when this type of inflammation is reported?

194 What non-surgical method can be tried to remove a subcutaneous bot fly?

193 i. 1 = infundibulum; 2 = isthmus; 3 = inferior segment; 4 = arrector pili muscle; 5 = sebaceous gland; 6 = epitrichial (sweat) gland; 7 = inner root sheath; 8 = outer root sheath; 9 = dermal papilla. This is a primary hair. Although secondary hairs can have associated sebaceous glands, only primary hairs will have an arrector pili muscle and an epitrichial (sweat) gland.

ii. Anagen is the phase of active growth where hair shafts are produced. This is followed by catagen, the phase of regression. During catagen there is cessation of mitotic activity of the matrix cells as well as apoptosis in the inferior portion of the hair follicle. Telogen is the resting phase of the hair follicle, when the inner root sheath is replaced by trichilemmal keratin and is reduced to about one-third of its former length; the hair is retained in the follicle as a dead hair.

iii. Luminal folliculitis is inflammation of the hair follicle with involvement of the follicular lumen. This pattern is the most commonly recognized type of follicular inflammation and is characterized by the presence of intraluminal inflammatory cells, typically neutrophils and/or eosinophils. Luminal folliculitis begins as mural folliculitis or inflammation of the wall of the hair follicle. However, in mural folliculitis, the inflammatory cells remain within the wall of the hair follicle and do not invade the hair follicle lumen. Differentials include bacterial folliculitis or furunculosis, dermatophytosis, demodicosis, sterile eosinophilic pustulosis, *Pelodera* nematodes, and sterile eosinophilic pinnal folliculitis.

194 The goal of treatment is to remove the bot fly. Spontaneous extrusion can occur and can also be 'encouraged'. Occlusion of the central pore with petroleum jelly, oil, or honey may trigger the parasite to back out of the hole. This 'home remedy' has been used in people with success and by one of the authors for a bot fly located in the medial canthus of a kitten. Surgical removal is the most commonly used technique for *Cuterebra* larvae removal. Surgical extraction requires making a large enough incision to extract the organism without damaging it. It can be difficult to extract bot fly larvae because their surface spines anchor them to surrounding tissue. Careful removal is important because any remaining tissue from the larva can cause an intense foreign body reaction. Anecdotal reports of anaphylaxis during removal have been reported.

195 In dogs, three species of *Demodex* mites have been identified. *D. canis* is the most common species of *Demodex* in the dog; these mites live in hair follicles, may cause localized or generalized disease, and may present in either juvenile- or adult-onset scenarios. *D. cornei* is a short-bodied mite that lives in the most superficial layer of the epidermis (stratum corneum); this mite has only been reported as a concurrent infestation with *D. canis*.
i. What is the third species of *Demodex* mite reported in the dog?
ii. Where does this mite reside in relation to the skin?
iii. How does the disease present clinically?
iv. What breed of dog has this been reported in most commonly?

196 A 12-year-old male castrated German shepherd-cross dog presented for multifocal raised erythematous masses. The owners reported that these lesions had been present for the past several years and previous treatments (several courses of systemic antibiotics, topical corticosteroids, bathing) did not appear beneficial. The lesions seemed to wax and wane; however, the owners felt more nodules had developed over the past

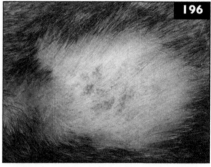

few years. The masses did not appear to cause the dog discomfort; they were neither painful nor pruritic and the dog appeared to otherwise be in good general health. On physical examination, multifocal to coalescing raised, erythematous nodules were noted along the dorsum, trunk, and lateral aspects of the hindlimbs (**196**). The lesions were firm and a bit waxy on the surface.
i. Based solely on the clinical appearance, what are the differential diagnoses for this patient?
ii. The pathologist reports a nodular to diffuse granulomatous reaction, but comments that lymphocytes are oddly missing. Of your differential diagnoses, and considering the history, what disease is most suspect?

195 i. *Demodex injai* (195).

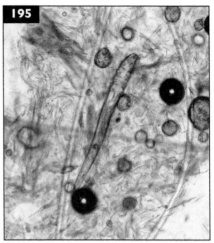

ii. This mite also lives in hair follicles; however, it occupies the space from the follicular opening to the level of and including the sebaceous glands.

iii. Although this mite does not appear to be common, it seems to be associated with dorsal greasy seborrhea. Erythema and scaling may also be present. Pruritus is variably present. Sebaceous hyperplasia may be a concurrent feature.

iv. Wire-haired fox terriers; in general, terrier breeds may be predisposed to this mite. Ivermectin (0.3–0.4 mg/kg q24h for 2–7 months) has been reported to be effective for treatment of *D. injai* as indicated by two consecutive negative skin scrapes.

196 i. Infectious (bacterial including deep pyoderma, atypical bacterial infection with *Mycobacteria*, *Nocardia*, *Actinomyces*, L-form infection, botryomycosis; fungal including dermatophytic mycetoma, blastomycosis, histoplasmosis, coccidioidomycosis, cryptococcosis, sporotrichosis), non-infectious inflammatory (reactive histiocytosis, sterile granuloma/pyogranuloma syndrome, sarcoidosis), neoplasia (multiple follicular tumors, cutaneous lymphoma, mast cell tumor, hamartoma).

ii. Sarcoidosis, a nodular inflammatory disease of uncertain etiology. In people, it is thought that the disease may be related to mycobacterial infections (particular tuberculosis) since mycobacterial DNA has been identified in granulomatous sarcoidosis lesions. Histopathology of the lesions lacks the lymphocytic component that is noted with other granulomatous skin diseases; they are often described as 'naked' granulomas due to this appearance of biopsy specimens. Lesions are described as multifocal granulomas composed of epithelioid macrophages without a peripheral accumulation of lymphocytes and without peripheral palisading. The disease to date has been reported in people, horses, and dogs. Human and equine sarcoidosis may be noted to have systemic organ involvement; to date, only the cutaneous form of the disease has been reported in dogs.

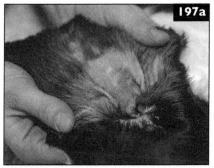
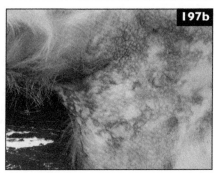

197 A 10-year-old male castrated English springer spaniel dog presented for multiple erythematous skin lesions. The owner reported that the dog had a several year history of waxing and waning non-pruritic lesions that had increased in severity over the past 2 years. On clinical examination, there were multifocal erythematous plaques on the concave surfaces of both pinnae (197a), the external ear canals, the ventral abdominal, and the preputial and perineal regions (197b). Several smaller erythematous papules were noted in the same regions. The plaques had a corrugated and somewhat waxy-scaly surface.

i. What are the differential diagnoses for this patient?

ii. Biopsy results showed an irregularly acanthotic epidermis with several deep projections (rete ridges) into the dermis and focal areas of parakeratosis, several intraepidermal pustules containing eosinophils and neutrophils, and mild dermal lichenoid inflammation composed of predominantly lymphocytes and plasma cells. Given this description, what is your most likely diagnosis?

iii. What is known or suspected about the pathogenesis of this condition?

198 A 2-year-old female spayed West Highland white terrier dog, recently diagnosed with AD, is receiving subcutaneous allergen immunotherapy. The dog has completed the induction phase of therapy and the owners have re-ordered the maintenance vial. The dog is receiving 1.0 ml of allergen (20,000 PNUs/ml) subcutaneously once every 7 days. The owners report that the dog is pruritic for approximately 24 hours after receiving the allergen. The pruritus is focal at first, but after a few hours the dog exhibits more widespread pruritus involving all four paws. What are the options for making the dog more comfortable?

197 i. Lichenoid dermatosis, primary seborrhea, actinic keratosis, atypical presentation of bacterial pyoderma, allergic skin disease.
ii. Psoriasiform-lichenoid dermatosis.
iii. This rare disease, typified by erythematous plaque lesions that are non-pruritic, most frequently affects the anatomic locations described in this case. The condition is most common in English springer spaniel dogs; breed predilection suggests a genetic/heritability component with regard to pathogenesis. The exact etiology is not known. The condition was first described in 1986. It has since been proposed that the condition may represent a distinctive reaction to superficial staphylococcal infection, possibly genetically programed. A case series described similar lesions in three dogs treated with cyclosporine for various inflammatory skin disorders, although these dogs were not spaniels. Although the lesions share similar characteristics on histopathology, psoriasiform-lichenoid dermatosis is not a true counterpart to psoriasis in humans. Although it is suspected to have a genetic component, psoriasiform-lichenoid dermatosis is not an immune-mediated condition, as is noted in people. The lesions in this dog responded well to treatment with oral antibiotics (doxycycline, 5 mg/kg q12h) for 30 days plus topical bathing with an antimicrobial shampoo as maintenance; at recheck, plaques were not present and only mild lacy hyperpigmentation remained. (**Note:** This disease does not appear to be as common as was once described in the literature. This may be due to breeders actively removing affected individuals or other unknown factors.)

198 Includes reducing the volume of allergens injected (often to a known volume that did not cause any adverse effects), increasing the number of days between injections, adding oral antihistamine therapy or low-dose glucocorticoid therapy, or adding in topical treatments (e.g. glucocorticoid sprays, antipruritic shampoos). The best option for this patient would be to start with a lower volume of allergen mixture per injection by either reducing the injection volume to the last volume at which the dog did not react, or decreasing the volume by 25% if the client cannot remember. If the dog continues to have 'flares' involved with immunotherapy administration, the volume of allergen can be reduced by decrements of 25% until the dog is comfortable, with the plan then slowly to attempt increased volumes. In some cases it is not the volume of allergen that is problematic, but the interval between injections. In most patients the interval is eventually increased to every 14–21 days. Successful immunotherapy with longer intervals is uncommon. An indication that the interval between injections needs to be shortened is a patient that is doing well but becomes pruritic shortly after the allergen injection. Management of allergy patients receiving immunotherapy via injections often requires changes in the volume of allergen being administered per injection, the time between injections, or both.

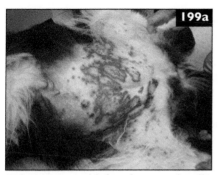
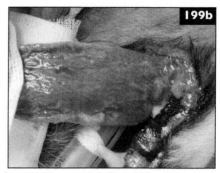

199 A 5-year-old female spayed collie dog was presented for the problems of depression, anorexia, and drooling. Physical examination revealed mild periocular erythema and hair loss, mucocutaneous ulcerations, oral ulcers and vesicles extending into the caudal pharynx, and ulcerative annular and serpiginous lesions in the axillary and inguinal regions (199a, b). The owner reported that the dog had been depressed and intermittently anorexic for the last 2 weeks.
i. What are possible differential diagnoses?
ii. Skin biopsy revealed the following: lymphocytic interface dermatitis and folliculitis with vesiculation at the dermal–epidermal junction. What is the diagnosis, and how is this condition treated?

200 A 5-year-old male castrated retired racing greyhound dog was presented for lameness on all four paws, but worse on the forepaws. Examination revealed several circumscribed areas of hyperkeratosis located centrally on multiple digital pads (200). Palpation of the lesions was painful.
i. What is this lesion?
ii. What is the etiology?
iii. Describe the histologic features of this condition.
iv. How is this treated or managed?

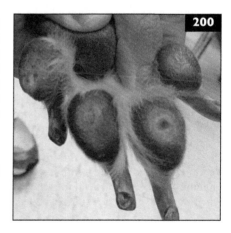

199 i. Bullous pemphigoid, pemphigus vulgaris, paraneoplastic pemphigus, SLE, EM, drug reaction, TEN, neoplasia, opportunistic infection, resistant bacterial infection.
ii. VCLE (of collie dogs and Shetland sheepdogs). This is not a new disease; in fact, the disease and its breed predilection have long been reported in the literature by various names. When the disease was first described in the early 1970s it was termed 'hidradenitis suppurativa' with a known breed predilection for collies, Shetland sheepdogs, and their crosses. In the early 1980s it was reclassified as a clinical variant of bullous pemphigoid. Over time this disease was renamed 'idiopathic ulcerative dermatosis of collies and Shetland sheepdogs'. The current name change to VCLE represents findings that support this disease as being a variant of CLE. There is some evidence that this disease may be exacerbated by sunlight and affected individuals often have lesions that worsen in the summer months and regress in the winter. Routine ANA tests are negative, but specialized testing has identified autoantibodies. This disease waxes and wanes and durable remission can be difficult to obtain. Corticosteroids are frequently utilized in management of the disease, typically at immunosuppressive doses. Cyclosporine may be an option in some dogs. Depending on the location of the lesions, topical tacrolimus or potentiated glucocorticoids may be used. Sun avoidance is recommended.

200 i. Paw-pad keratoma (paw-pad corn, or callus). Synonyms include keratoderma, tyloma, and tylosis.
ii. This lesion occurs almost exclusively in racing or retired greyhound dogs and other related sight hounds. Evidence supports a mechanical etiology; weight-bearing digits on the forelimbs appear to be most commonly affected, supporting the influence of repeated trauma, particularly during racing. Foreign body penetration may also lead to corn formation; surgical exploration and diagnostic imaging (e.g. radiography) have found imbedded plant material, metal, and grit within various corn lesions in greyhounds.
iii. Lesions are typically characterized by well-demarcated, dome-shaped, conical or cylindrical mounds of compact hyperkeratosis. The keratin projects above the skin surface and frequently also extends downwards, forming a depression in the epidermis, a feature unique to paw-pad keratoma. Exaggerated digitated surface configuration (rete ridge formation) is also typically noted on histopathology. In most cases, inflammation is mild to absent unless acute trauma or fissuring is evident.
iv. Surgical excision is the treatment of choice for paw-pad corns; however, the rate of recurrence is fairly high. Techniques include laser removal, physical extrusion, curettage, and removal of the firm center. Soft padded bandages or boots may minimize further trauma to the area. Distal digital ostectomy (removal of the distal phalanx) has been beneficial in some cases; however, this may not prove favorable when multiple digits on multiple paws are involved.

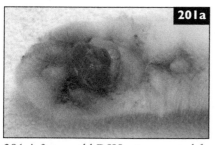
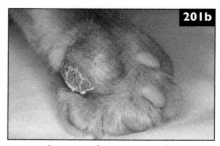

201 A 3-year-old DSH cat presented for a 1-year history of progressive lameness. The cat lived indoors and there were no other cats in the home. Physical examination was normal except for lesions on the foot pads (**201a**). Large ulcerative masses were present on both front paws. The owner had reported that when the lameness first started the foot pads were soft and 'puffy' (**201b**). The foot pad lesions waxed and waned, often becoming ulcerative.

i. Cytologic aspirate of a foot pad revealed a mixed inflammatory infiltrate with plasma cells. A skin biopsy was obtained and was consistent with feline plasma cell pododermatitis (PCD). Although the history and physical examination findings alone were highly suggestive of PCD, at the time of presentation, this disease presents with a wide range of clinical signs. What other differential diagnoses need to be ruled out?

ii. What are the common clinical characteristics of this disease, and what is known about the etiology?

202 A 6-year-old rough coated collie dog presents with acute severe pruritus of the entire ventrum. Pruritic, alopecic, and erythematous regions include the elbows and the margins of the ear pinnae. You perform skin scrapes, which are negative for mites. The owner notes that the dog spends about 50% of its time outside and that he has seen foxes in the area lately. The owner reports that recently he has developed

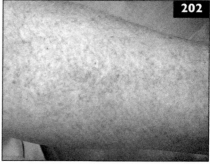

a pruritic rash, and in fact lifts his shirt up to show you that it is mainly on his abdomen and forearms (**202**).

i. Based on your strong suspicion, you elect to treat empirically for what disease?

ii. What treatment options are available for this dog? What concerns do you have related to the breed of dog and the possible treatments?

201 i. Pemphigus, lupus erythematosus, chemical or physical trauma, infection or sterile pyogranuloma, eosinophilic lesions, neoplasia (mastocytoma, lympho-sarcoma), foreign body reaction.

ii. PCD has only been reported in cats and there is no recognized sex, breed, or age predilection. The etiology is unknown, but it has very characteristic clinical manifestations. It begins as a soft spongy swelling on one, but usually on multiple foot pads, with the central carpal and metarsal foot pads most commonly affected. In some cases the foot pads will have a violaceous color and may have striations present (see **197b**). Pain is variable with the initial foot pad swelling. Most cats are asymptomatic for a long period of time, but usually become lame once lesions become ulcerative. Large ulcerated proliferative masses, as occurred in this case, are not typical. Cats can present with concurrent plasma cell stomatitis or swellings on the bridge of their nose and nasal planum. A hypergammaglobulinemia (polyclonal gammopathy), tissue infiltration with plasma cells, and response to immunomodulatory drugs strongly support an immune-mediated etiology. In one study, several of the cats were FIV positive, but the relationship between PCD and FIV is yet unknown. PCD may be a reaction pattern to a yet unidentified antigen, as there has been at least one report of plasma cell infiltrate causing nasal swelling in a cat without concurrent paw lesions.

202 i. *Sarcoptes scabiei.*
ii. Weekly dips with 2–3% lime sulfur are very effective. Other treatment options include milbemycin oxime, selamectin, moxidectin, ivermectin, and topical fipronil. Treatment should continue for two complete life cycles of the mite (6 weeks total). Amitraz dips are also effective, but may be associated with sedation, ataxia, and bradycardia. While systemic treatment options are very effective, there is particular concern with the use of avermectins in collies. Collie dogs that are homozygous for a mutation in the *ABCB1* gene (also known as the *MDR1* gene) accumulate high levels of ivermectin in the CNS. Ivermectin is a macrocyclic lactone. This class of drugs works through potentiation of GABA-gated chloride ion channels. GABA-gated chloride channels exist throughout the peripheral nervous system of arthropods and nematodes, and potentiation of them causes inhibition of neurologic activity. In mammals, GABA-gated channels exist only within the CNS. The *ABCB1* gene encodes P-glycoprotein, a transmembrane protein pump that is responsible for the efflux of xenobiotics from the intracellular space and is a major component of the blood–brain barrier. The majority of collie dogs carry at least one copy of a deletion mutation (nt228[del4])in the *ABCB1* gene. Dogs that are homozygous for this mutation are unable to efflux ivermectin and experience neurotoxicity at low doses of ivermectin (0.1 mg/kg). Affected collies may also be more susceptible to neurotoxicity with other macrocyclic lactones (e.g. milbemycin, selamectin, moxidectin), although studies have shown that selamectin and moxidectin have wide safety profiles even in ivermectin-sensitive collies. PCR testing for the nt228(del4) gene mutation is available.

203 A 12-year-old female spayed mixed-breed dog presented for severe, acute swelling of both pinnae. The owner reported that the dog had been shaking her head frequently for the past 2 days; the swelling was noted only on the day of presentation.

i. Given the history, clinical description of the ear, and acute presentation, what is the most likely diagnosis for this patient?

ii. What diagnostic tests and treatment options should be recommended?

iii. Although there can be several causes, what is the most common underlying cause for this condition?

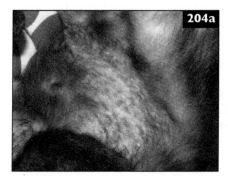 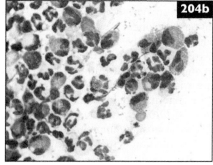

204 The ventral abdomen of a 5-year-old cat is shown (**204a**). The lesion has been treated repeatedly with methylprednisolone acetate (20 mg/cat SC). Initially, the lesion resolved for 3–6 months, but recently the interval between lesion recurrence has decreased to 1–2 months. Close inspection of the lesion reveals that it is intensely pruritic (cat observed to self-traumatize lesion), erosive, exudative, and raised. Further dermatologic examination reveals blunted whiskers, hair loss on the chin, mild ceruminous otitis externa, and scaling on the hair coat. Skin scrapings, flea combings, and dermatophyte culture are negative. Impression smears of the lesion are shown (**204b**).

i. What is the clinical diagnosis of this lesion?

ii. How is this lesion treated?

Answers: 203, 204

203 i. Aural hematoma.

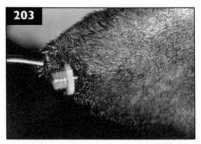

ii. Drainage and repair of the hematoma should be discussed with the owner. Numerous options exist: surgical correction, cannulation (**203**), suction drain placement, punch biopsy technique, and laser technique. The prognosis is good for any of the treatment options. If drainage is not accomplished, the hematoma will eventually coagulate and organize making surgical repair much more difficult. Scarring is a common side-effect of untreated aural hematomas. Ear swab cytology should be performed to evaluate organisms in the ear canal. Otoscopic evaluation should also be performed.

iii. Otitis externa. This may be due to any of several factors including allergic disease, endocrinopathies, parasites, neoplasia, foreign body, or cornification defects. Secondary bacterial and/or yeast overgrowth are/is commonly noted. These should be diagnosed and treated accordingly. Otitis externa should be managed aggressively to aid the healing of aural hematomas; oral prednisone or prednisolone may be administered for the first few days to reduce inflammation. If ear infections and/or aural hematomas are recurrent, the underlying etiology of otitis externa should be identified and a long-term management plan formulated. In cats, *Otodectes* infestation is the most common underlying etiology; allergic disease is most common in dogs. Underlying allergies are commonly overlooked as a cause of aural hematomas in dogs.

204 i. Eosinophilic plaque.

ii. Eosinophilic plaques are now recognized to be the 'hot spots' of cats with a similar pathogenesis. An intensely pruritic event initiates self-trauma at a focal area, which rapidly becomes exudative, creating an 'itch–scratch' trigger. Secondary bacterial and yeast colonization are very common and underrecognized complicating factors contributing to the pruritus. Impression smears of these lesions may reveal predominantly eosinophilic inflammation with intracellular and/or extracellular bacteria and yeast. This is in contrast to what is seen in cases of canine pyoderma, in which neutrophilic exudate predominates. Treatment for the lesion alone includes a 21–30-day course of antibiotics (potentiated sulfa antibiotics, cephalosporins, clindamycin). If yeast are present, itraconazole, fluconazole, or terbinafine can be administered and/or the cat can be treated with a topical antibacterial/antifungal shampoo. Many cats with these lesions will respond to antibiotic therapy alone. Topical antimicrobial therapy may be beneficial if the cat will tolerate it.

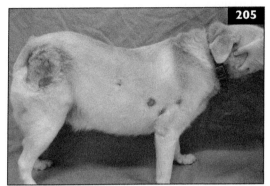

205 A 7-year-old male neutered yellow Labrador retriever dog presents with multiple, partially alopecic, raised, freely moveable, non-adhered, palpably fluctuant nodules with associated draining tracts on the trunk (205). Lesions have been present for 2 weeks. The owner reports lesions quickly develop and come to a 'head', after which they drain with a glossy yellow-brown material. Nodules are painful to the touch. The dog is moderately depressed, slightly febrile, and has generalized peripheral lymphadenopathy. However, the owner reports the dog is eating, drinking, urinating, and defecating normally. Cytologic impression smears of exudate from the lesions do not reveal bacteria or yeast.
i. List the differential diagnoses for these draining nodular lesions.
ii. What diagnostic tests are needed to confirm the diagnosis?
iii. What is the most probable diagnosis given the character of the oily discharge?

206 Glucocorticoid administration has been associated with what life-threatening side-effect in cats?

Answers: 205, 206

205 i. Inflammatory/infectious (deep staphylococcal pyoderma, nocardiosis, actinomycosis, L-form bacteriosis, mycobacteriosis, subcutaneous mycoses), inflammatory/non-infectious (foreign body, cutaneous/follicular cyst, sterile nodular panniculitis, histiocytic disease), and neoplasia.
ii. Deep incisional or excisional wedge biopsies of nodules for histopathology and culture. If possible, select nodules with an intact surface epithelium to avoid superficial microbial contamination. Special stains (e.g. PAS, GMS, acid-fast) and polarized light examination of tissue should be requested to exclude microorganisms and foreign bodies, respectively. Fine-needle aspirate cytology of nodules can be misleading depending on the developmental stage of the nodule.
iii. Sterile nodular panniculitis (SNP). The nature of the discharge is suggestive of saponification of the panniculus. Adipose tissue is fragile and prone to traumatic, ischemic, and inflammatory insults. Injury to lipocytes causes release of lipids, which are degraded into inflammation-inducing free fatty acids. Consequently, an oxidative inflammatory cascade results in a pyogranulomatous to granulomatous tissue response. Panniculitis has been associated with physicochemical factors (trauma, injections, foreign bodies), infections, nutritional disorders (vitamin E deficiency), immunologic conditions (lupus), and pancreatic disorders (inflammation, neoplasia). When a specific etiology cannot be identified, the disease is termed SNP; infectious agents must be ruled out because treatment for SNP involves immunosuppressive/immunomodulatory agents.

206 Congestive heart failure (CHF). Glucocorticoids, particularly methyl-prednisolone acetate, can be a trigger for the development of CHF in cats with 'compensated or asymptomatic' hypertrophic cardiomyopathy. In one study CHF developed within 1–19 days of administration of glucocorticoids in a small number of cases. In approximately half of the cats in this report, CHF was cured and morphologic cardiac changes partially or completely resolved. The temporal association between corticosteroid administration, the initial diagnosis of CHF, and the clinical course of the disease suggests that this may be a unique form of CHF called 'corticosteroid-associated CHF'. Overall this condition is rare.

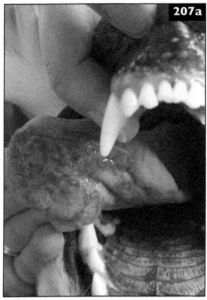

207 A 5-year-old male intact golden retriever dog presented for halitosis, excessive salivation, and difficulty eating. The owners had noticed multiple masses along the gingiva and tongue within 2 days of presentation (207a). The dog was otherwise feeling fairly well. The owners reported no decrease in his energy during a hunting trip the previous weekend.
i. What are your differentials for this patient?
ii. What diagnostic tests what would you recommend for this dog?

208 i. What are bacteriophages?
ii. What is their potential for use?
iii. What is known about their use in veterinary dermatology?

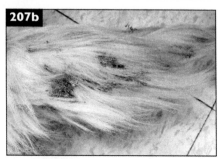

207 i. The lesions appear to be proliferative to nodular with ulceration frequently covered by a mucoid, membranous layer. Differentials should include those for both nodules (infections – including deep fungal mycoses, opportunistic fungal infections, bacterial, viral; inflammatory – foreign body reaction, chemical or thermal burn injury; neoplasia – amelanotic melanoma, SCC, soft tissue sarcoma) and necrotizing diseases (drug eruption, foreign body reaction, chemical or thermal burn, immune-mediated diseases – lupus, pemphigus vulgaris).
ii. Biopsy would allow for identification of any neoplastic or possibly infectious etiology. Tissue culture may be indicated to confirm or refute the presence of an infectious organism. In this dog, a more thorough history and physical examination were obtained. There was no history of previous medications, making drug eruption an unlikely diagnosis. No history of burn or chemical insult was apparent. The owner again mentioned the hunting trip the weekend prior to presentation. On closer examination, several prickly heads of a Burdock plant (burrs) were found stuck throughout the tail and fur of the feet (207b). Sedated examination of the oral cavity revealed numerous fine burr particles embedded throughout the lesions on the tongue and gingiva. Foreign body granuloma was confirmed on biopsy. Surgical debridement and removal of the burrs from the dog's coat led to complete resolution.

208 i. Viruses that infect bacterial organisms. Subsequently, they can potentially kill and lyse the bacteria they infect, but do not kill or infect cells belonging to humans or animals.
ii. Bacteriophages have been beneficial for the treatment of various bacterial diseases; the use of bacteriophages is a potential intervention for treatment of multidrug-resistant bacteria.
iii. Two studies evaluated the use of bacteriophage therapy for *Pseudomonas* otitis externa in dogs, and the results were promising. Treatment with bacteriophages for cutaneous burns has also been documented in a mouse model; the possibility for translation to other animal species exists.

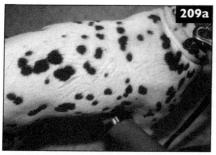
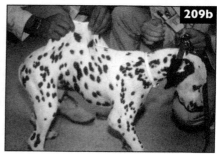

209 A 6-month-old dog presented with linear white scars (**209a**) on the trunk. There was no history of excessive trauma. Close examination of the scars revealed atrophic irregular tissue that was easily torn. The dog also had a history of chronic hygroma formation on the elbows (note lesion on the right forelimb [**209b**]). The skin was hyperextensible (**209b**).
i. What is the difference between cutaneous asthenia, dermatosparaxis, and Ehlers–Danlos syndrome (EDS)?
ii. What is the diagnosis in this patient?
iii. What other clinical signs commonly occur in this disease?
iv. How do you confirm the diagnosis?

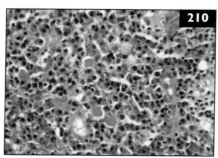

210 A 4-year-old male castrated DSH cat presented with an acute swelling on the nose. The owner reported that the lesion had developed over the last week. Physical examination was otherwise normal.
i. Biopsy of the nose is shown (**210**). What is the diagnosis for this cat?
ii. What treatment options may be considered for this patient?

209 i. Cutaneous asthenia describes disorders that involve both collagen and elastin. Dermatosparaxis describes disorders caused by a type I procollagen-N-peptidase mutation. EDS is a heterogenous group of connective tissue disorders characterized by reduced tensile strength of affected tissue. The latter is recognized by skin hyperextensibility, joint hypermobility, and tissue fragility.
ii. EDS, a heritable disease. Spontaneous disease occurrence has been reported in people, rabbits, dogs, cats, horses, and cattle. In dogs and cats, both dominant and recessive forms of inheritance occur.
iii. Widening of the bridge of the nose, subcutaneous hematomas, elbow hygromas, hernias, joint laxity, microcornea, sclerocornea, lens luxation, cataracts.
iv. History and clinical signs; diagnosis by biopsy can be difficult as tissue can appear normal. When changes are present, histologic findings include alterations in arrangement, length, and staining characteristics of collagen fibers. Masson's trichrome stain will show abnormalities of collagen. There is no effective treatment for this disease; control focuses primarily on managing symptoms. As the skin is easily torn, care must be taken to prevent/minimize secondary infections. Delayed wound healing is problematic. People report significant joint pain, joint dislocations, muscle cramps, fatigue, and headache. Because of the rarity of the disease in animals, little is known about the quality of life of affected dogs and cats. Breeding from these animals is not recommended.

210 i. Plasma cell infiltrate. There is marked perivascular to diffuse dermal infiltration with plasma cells, occasional Mott cells, and small lymphocytes. A few neutrophils are also present. Feline plasma cell pododermatitis commonly presents with this same histopathology finding; however, plasma cell infiltrate has also been reported in a cat with nasal lesions in the absence of paw-pad disease.
ii. The exact pathogenesis of this condition in cats is not known, but the presence of plasma cells, hypergammaglobulinemia on serum chemistry analysis, and response to treatment are suggestive of an immune-mediated etiology. The condition is generally responsive to corticosteroid administration. Prednisolone (4 mg/kg q24h) is generally needed to induce remission; response is typically seen within 2–3 weeks of starting therapy, at which time the dose should be reduced. Doxycycline has also been shown to be beneficial in most cats with this disease; 5–10 mg/kg q12–24h typically brings resolution within 1–2 months. Oral suspension should be administered due to the potential for esophageal stricture with this medication. Cyclosporine (5–10 mg/kg q24h) is another option for treatment; most cats respond well. In some patients, treatment may be discontinued following resolution without relapse in clinical signs. Other patients require life long treatment to maintain remission.

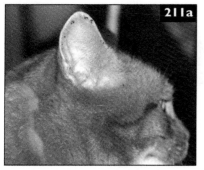
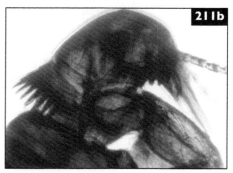

211 A cat was presented for the complaint of 'itchy twitchy ears'. Close inspection of the ears revealed these small black specks (**211a**).
i. This organism was removed from the cat's ear (**211b**). Identify this parasite.
ii. What is the natural host, and how did the cat acquire this organism?

212 A four-year-old female spayed pug dog presents for chronic ear infection of several weeks' duration. Until this event, the dog had no prior history of skin disease. Physical examination reveals a large amount of ceruminous debris in both external canals (**212**). Otoscopic examination is attempted; however, the canal lumen is extremely stenotic, less than 25% of the normal diameter. As can be seen in the image,

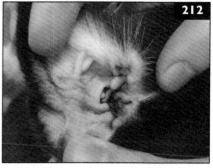

there is a large amount of redundant folding near the canal opening. Palpation of the ear canals is painful to the dog; both canals feel thickened. The remainder of the physical examination is normal, except for an excessive amount of exfoliated scale along the body. The owner reports that this has been a historic finding for the dog, but has not prompted her to seek treatment.
i. What is the likely primary cause of this dog's chronic ear infections?
ii. What is the progression of ear disease in these patients?
iii. What dog breeds are predisposed to this problem?

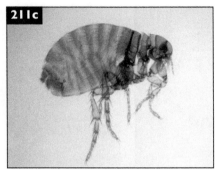

211 i. *Spilopsyllus cuniculi* (European rabbit flea). It is differentiated from cat and dog fleas by the almost vertical position of its genal comb and rounded ends of the spines, compared with the horizontal position and sharp points found on *Ctenocephalides felis* (**211c**).
ii. Rabbits. It is acquired by cats or dogs from rabbit burrows. It can cause severe irritation on the pinnae of cats. It can also carry and transmit myxomatosis.

212 i. A cornification disorder. This is supported by the proliferative tissue in the ears as well as the excessive scaling along the rest of the dog's coat.
ii. Failure of epithelial migration begins the process of external ear canal pathology. This creates an increased amount of debris in the canal (cerumen, exfoliated skin cells) as self-cleaning is impaired. Edema formation follows, which allows for increased moisture in the canals. The combination of increased humidity and debris serves as an ideal environment for microbial overgrowth. Glandular hyperplasia further increases the ceruminous debris present. Redundant folding follows, giving the ear canal the appearance of corrugated cardboard. The combination of edema and redundant folding can markedly decrease the canal diameter, causing stenosis. The tissue may eventually become fibrotic, followed by calcification/ossification. This is indicative of end-stage ear disease. At this point, medical management is not possible.
iii. Spaniel breeds in general, particularly cocker spaniel and springer spaniel dogs. West Highland white terrier and Bassett hound dogs are also commonly affected.

213 A 2-year-old male castrated cocker spaniel dog was presented for progressive alopecia, erythema, and crusting of the periocular skin bilaterally (213). The owner reported mild facial pruritus. The only other medical problem was a prior diagnosis of keratoconjunctivitis sicca for which the dog has been receiving topical eye drops. No other dermatologic abnormalities were identified on physical examination other than the bilaterally symmetrical periocular alopecia, erythema, and crusting.

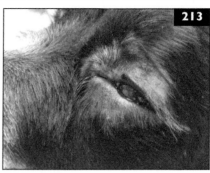

i. Based on the clinical appearance of the lesions, what differential diagnoses should be considered?
ii. What initial diagnostic tests should be recommended?

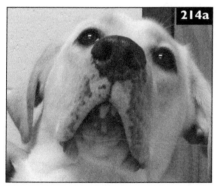
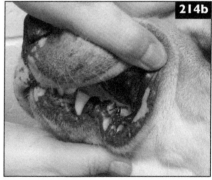

214 A 9-month-old male castrated Labrador retriever dog presented for mild swelling, erythema, and depigmentation along the front of the muzzle (214a) and lips (214b) of approximately 2 weeks' duration. The dog was otherwise healthy. Physical examination did not reveal any other abnormal findings. No other mucous membranes or haired skin were affected other than what is shown.

i. What additional questions should be asked of the owner with regard to the history and progression of the disease?
ii. What are your differential diagnoses for this patient? What initial diagnostic tests are indicated?

213 i. Dermatophytosis, demodicosis, allergic skin disease (including cutaneous adverse reaction to food and AD), drug reaction, PF, ocular discomfort leading to secondary trauma to the periocular skin.

ii. Wood's lamp evaluation and DTM culture should be performed for dermatophytes. Deep skin scraping and/or hair plucks should be obtained to look for *Demodex* mites. Cytologic evaluation of the skin should be carried out to look for microbial overgrowth. A repeat Schirmer tear test and ocular examination should be performed to determine if the cause of the discomfort is ocular. Depending on the findings of these core diagnostic tests, skin biopsy may be necessary to obtain a definitive diagnosis.

In this case, all core dermatologic diagnostics tests were negative. On questioning the owner further, she reported that the dog's cyclosporine ophthalmic ointment had been changed several weeks prior to the skin lesion development. The medication had been compounded in a corn oil base as opposed to the dog's normal aqueous drops. Reformulation of the medication into an aqueous base resulted in complete resolution of the dermatologic abnormalities.

214 i. What is the dog's vaccination history? What other medications are being administered, either by prescription or over the counter? What is the dog's environment? What toys, dishes, blankets, or other objects come into contact with the dog's mouth and face? Are other animals affected? Has there been any remodeling in the home? Does anyone have any hobbies that involve volatile chemicals? Is the dog pruritic? What about littermates?

ii. Include early stages of juvenile cellulitis (lack of lymph node swelling and signs of systemic illness would make this less likely), contact irritation, and drug reaction. Although this is not a commonly affected breed and the dog is very young, uveodermatologic syndrome should also be considered, although it is fairly unlikely. Because of this possibility, a thorough ocular examination should be part of the initial diagnostic evaluation. Other tests include cytology, dermatophyte culture, skin scrapings, and possible biopsy. In this case, the owner mentioned that the dog had been given a new rubber ball to play with shortly before clinical signs developed. After removing all other rubber toys and the new ball, clinical signs resolved completely; contact irritation/hypersensitivity was diagnosed.

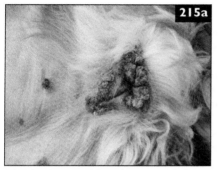
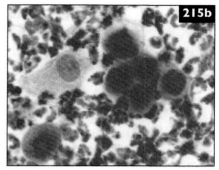

215 A 13-year-old cocker spaniel dog presented for a history of excessive crusting and lameness. The dog also was noted to have been febrile for the past month and more lethargic than usual. Treatment for presumed Lyme's disease (doxycycline) had been prescribed by the primary care veterinarian approximately 3 weeks prior to presentation. On questioning the owners, they reported that the dog had always been excessively scaly and had an oily coat; however, crusting seemed to have increased markedly within the past 2 weeks. On physical examination, thick mounded crusts were present on the nasal planum, foot pads of all four feet, concave surface of the pinnae, and around the vulva (**215a**). Similar crusted lesions were also present multifocally along the haired skin of the dorsum, ventrum, and flanks.

i. Given the history and physical examination findings, what are the differential diagnoses for this patient?

ii. Cytology from under a crusted skin lesion on the flank is shown (**215b**). What is the most likely diagnosis given this finding? What findings on a histopathology report would confirm the cytologic suspicion?

iii. What is the difference between drug-induced, drug-triggered, and naturally occurring PF?

216 i. What is IVIG?

ii. What is its proposed mechanism of action?

iii. What diseases has it been used to treat?

215 i. Primary disorder of keratinization (seborrhea), but does not explain the lethargy or lameness. The thick crusting along with lesions on the non-haired skin (foot pads, mucous membranes) increases suspicion of an autoimmune skin disease (particularly PF) or metabolic abnormality (superficial necrolytic dermatitis, zinc deficiency). Neoplasia (e.g. cutaneous lymphoma) would seem less likely given the symmetrical nature of the lesions; however, this should be considered in an older patient. The recent antibiotic administration would also add cutaneous drug eruption to the differential list.

ii. PF. Note the large numbers of acantholytic keratinocytes forming small groups or 'rafts' within a neutrophilic background. Histopathologic findings, including subcorneal pustules containing large numbers of neutrophils and acantholytic keratinocytes, support the diagnosis. Eosinophils may also be present in variable numbers. Infectious organisms would not be identified.

iii. Naturally occurring PF is the most common form of PF reported in domestic animal species; this form of the disease develops in the absence of any known trigger. Drug-induced PF mimics the natural disease, but it goes into remission with removal of the offending drug. Drug-triggered PF is also associated with drug administration, but does not go into remission with removal of the drug. It is suspected that the drug acts more to trigger the patient's natural predisposition towards development of PF. In dogs, this type of PF has most recently been associated with the administration of topical metaflumizone-amitraz.

216 i. Intravenous immunoglobulin. The current formulation is a highly purified infusion of human IgG antibodies.

ii. Suppression of inflammation by modulating the Th2 pathway. Other mechanisms of immunomodulation, although not fully understood, include neutralization of autoantibodies, inhibition of complement binding and activation, and suppression of pathogenic cytokines.

iii. In the dog, IVIG infusions have been used for the treatment of immune-mediated hemolytic anemia, cutaneous drug reactions, PF, and immune-mediated thrombocytopenia.

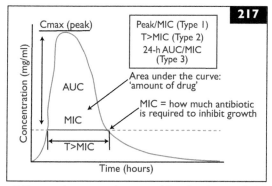

217i. What is the difference between pharmacokinetics (PK) and pharmacodynamics (PD) with respect to antibiotic therapy?

ii. Three PK parameters are used to quantify the activity of an antibiotic (**217**). Which ones are they, and how are they used to classify antibiotics when combined with MIC?

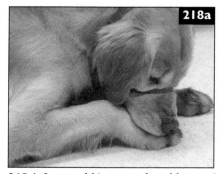

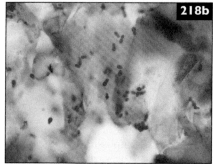

218 A 5-year-old intact male golden retriever dog presented for a history of chronic, non-seasonal pruritic dermatitis of approximately 3 years' duration. The owners felt that the severity of disease had been slowly progressive, but had remained confined to the feet. The dog was reported to be moderately pruritic, with a fair amount of time spent licking and chewing at his feet (**218a**). Salivary staining and moderate interdigital erythema was noted on both the dorsal and ventral aspects of all four feet.

i. An acetate tape impression of the feet is shown (**218b**). What are these organisms?

ii. With regard to treatment recommendations, what is the evidence for and against various options for control of this disease?

217 i. PK refers to the time course of antimicrobial concentrations in the body and PD to the relationship between those concentrations and the antimicrobial effect. MIC is an indicator of the potency of an antibiotic, but does not provide information about the time course of antibiotic activity.

ii. The three PK parameters that are most important are peak serum concentration (Cmax), trough serum concentration (Cmin), and the serum concentration time course (area under the curve [AUC]). When these are integrated with the MIC, the killing activity of antibiotics can be divided into time-dependent killing, concentration-dependent killing, and prolonged persistent effects. Antibiotics are classified into three general categories based on pattern of activity. Type I antibiotics (e.g. aminoglycosides, fluoroquinolones) are concentration dependent and therefore the goal of therapy is to have a dosing regimen that maximizes concentration, because the higher the concentration the more extensive and faster the degree of killing. The best predictors of this are the 24-hour AUC/MIC ratio and Cmax/MIC ratio. Type II antibiotics (e.g. beta-lactams, erythromycin, linezolid) have almost the opposite set of properties. The ideal dosing regimen is one that maximizes duration of exposure. The T>MIC (the percentage of time antimicrobial concentrations exceed the MIC) is the best predictor of this. For beta-lactams and erythromycin, maximum killing is seen when the time above the MIC is at least 70% of the dosing interval. Type III antibiotics (e.g. vancomycin, tetracycline, azithromycin) have mixed properties of time-dependent killing and moderate persistent effects. For these drugs the ideal dosing regimen maximizes the amount of drug received. The 24-hour AUC/MIC ratio is the parameter that correlates with efficacy.

218 i. *Malassezia* spp.; yeast organisms.

ii. Systematic reviews have evaluated various treatment options for *Malassezia* dermatitis in dogs. Based on the data, there is good evidence to recommend a sole topical treatment (2% miconazole nitrate and 2% chlorhexidine gluconate shampoo twice weekly for 3 weeks). Fair evidence exists for recommending oral ketoconazole (5–10 mg/kg q24h for 3 weeks) or oral itraconazole (5 mg/kg on 2 consecutive days of a week for 3 weeks), especially when topical treatment is impractical or impossible. There is insufficient evidence to recommend either oral terbinafine or various other topical treatments (miconazole, enilconazole, chlorhexidine, piroctone olamine, benzalkonium chloride) for treatment of *Malassezia* dermatitis in dogs. Although anecdotal reports exist with regard to other treatment options, more stringent and controlled studies need to be performed to further validate these therapeutic 'recommendations'.

219 A 6-year-old male castrated DSH cat presented for intense pruritus, exudative skin lesions, and progressive alopecia. The ventral abdomen was the most severely affected area (**219a**); however, the owner had also noted that the cat's lip appeared swollen. The cat spent 6 months of the year in Florida, USA, and the other 6 months in Wisconsin. No medications had been administered to the cat, including ectoparasite prevention.

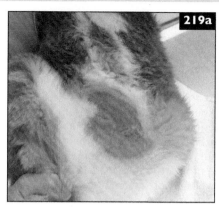

i. What are the differential diagnoses for the lesions seen on this cat?

ii. Cytology of the lesion on the ventral abdomen showed a large number of both eosinophils and neutrophils. Several coccoid bacteria, primarily in pairs or small clusters and often located intracellularly, were also seen. What are your treatment recommendations for this cat?

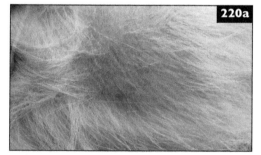

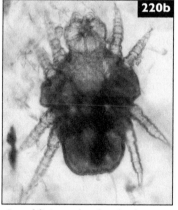

220 A 10-year-old mixed-breed dog treated for lymphoma developed mild to moderate pruritus, erythema, and excessive scaling over the last several months. The lesions shown were present extensively over the dorsum (**220a**). In addition, the dog had severe facial excoriations. Skin scrapings revealed large numbers of mites and eggs per high-power field (**220b**).

i. What is the diagnosis?

ii. What recommendations will you make to the ward staff?

219 i. Parasites (fleas, *Demodex gatoi*), infection (bacterial pyoderma, dermatophytosis), allergy (flea allergy dermatitis, cutaneous adverse reaction to food, environmental allergy). Abdominal and urinary tract pain would also be differentials for the lesions noted on the ventral abdomen.
ii. Since the cat is not currently receiving any ectoparasite prevention, initiating

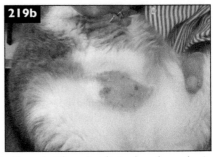

appropriate adulticide flea prevention is indicated. There is clinical and cytologic evidence of bacterial pyoderma, therefore appropriate antimicrobial therapy is recommended. Amoxicillin–clavulanate, cefadroxil, cefovecin, clindamycin, ormetoprim–sulfadimethoxine, or trimethoprim–sulfonamide are all effective for feline bacterial pyoderma. Based on response to the aforementioned treatments, a lime sulfur trial for *Demodex gatoi* and additional work-up for underlying allergic disease would be the next steps. This cat responded markedly to a single injection of cefovecin sodium and flea prevention using selamectin (**219b**). Repeated injection and maintenance of monthly flea prevention led to complete remission and no relapse of skin lesions.

220 i. *Cheyletiella* infestation. This is a severe infestation; it is uncommon to find large numbers of mites and eggs per high-power field. The mite causes dorsal scaling and mild to moderate pruritus in dogs, cats, and rabbits. The entire life cycle (approximately 35 days) is spent on the host. The mites do not burrow but rather move freely on the surface of the skin and deposit eggs on the hairs.
ii. This is a highly contagious disease and presents a risk to other dogs or cats housed in the ward that day. In this case, the risk is increased due to the large number of mites. Mites can live in the environment for short periods of time; they are very mobile. Transmission occurs via direct contact, environmental exposure, or by ward staff. If possible, move the dog to isolation. The cage and area where the dog was housed should be grossly cleaned and treated with an environmental insecticide labeled as effective against fleas. Ward staff need to be informed of the zoonotic risk and instructed to seek medical attention if they develop a pruritic rash. All staff should change their uniforms and laboratory coats and place them in a plastic bag until washed. Anyone handling the dog should wear gloves and disposable gowns. The owners need to be informed of the risk and educated about the treatment of their pet and other pets at home.

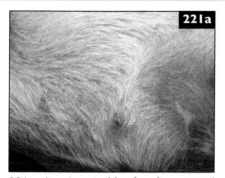

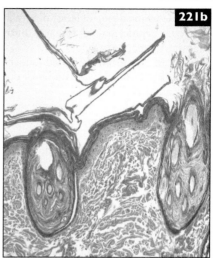

221 A 4-year-old female spayed Labrador retriever dog presented for excessive scaling and hair loss (221a). The owners had adopted the dog as a young adult; severe scaling was present at the time of adoption; however, it was attributed to poor nutrition since the dog was obtained from a rescue facility. The dog's clinical signs did not improve with antimicrobial therapy (systemic antibiotic administration) or corticosteroid administration. The owners reported the dog to be only mildly pruritic. On physical examination, large scales were present over the entire body with scaling worse along the limbs and trunk. The scales were tan–white in color and were either free in the hair coat or adhered to the skin in sheets. Hair loss was more noticeable in areas with excessive scaling. The skin beneath the exfoliative dermatitis was normal in appearance; ulcers and inflammation were absent. The nasal planum, foot pads, and mucocutaneous junctions were not affected.

i. What are the differential diagnoses for this patient?
ii. A skin biopsy from a region of excessive scale is shown (221b). What are the key findings?
iii. What is the diagnosis?
iv. What forms of this disease have been reported in the dog?

222 What options are there for environmental flea control (222)?

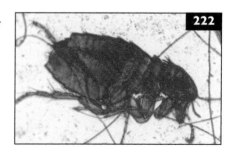

221 i. Cornification defect; differentials include severe primary seborrhea, ichthyosis, epidermal dysplasia, nutritional deficiency/responsive dermatosis (vitamin A, zinc, fatty acid).
ii. Marked compact/laminated superficial orthokeratotic hyperkeratosis and follicular keratosis; the remainder of the epidermis is of normal thickness. Dermal inflammation is not noted.
iii. Ichthyosis.
iv. Ichthyosis is used to describe a group of genetic skin diseases characterized by generalized scaling. The disease results from an abnormality in keratinocyte differentiation or cornification. The scaling is a result of either increased keratinocyte proliferation or decreased corneocyte desquamation. Although several forms of the disease exist in humans, only a few have been genetically characterized in the dog. All forms in the dog have been reported or suspected to be inherited as an autosomal recessive trait. A mutation in keratin 10 causes an epidermolytic form of ichthyosis in the Norfolk terrier. Non-epidermolytic forms of ichthyosis are more common in dogs. A mutation in transglutaminase-1 causes ichthyosis in Jack Russell terriers. In golden retriever dogs, genetic ichthyosis due to a PNPLA1 mutation associated with an autosomal recessive mode of inheritance has been reported. This disease is an animal model for human autosomal recessive congenital ichthyosis. Ichthyosis is also seen in other breeds of dogs; however, the genetic characterization has not yet been determined.

222 Mechanical removal of flea eggs and larvae can be done via regular and thorough vacuuming of the environment. Indoor environments can be sprayed with methoprene or pyriproxifen; these insect growth hormone analogs stop the development of flea eggs and larvae. Methoprene is degraded by UV light so it should only be used indoors. Pyriproxifen is more UV stable and can be used both indoors and outdoors; it remains in the environment for 2–4 months. Lufenuron is an insect development inhibitor that interferes with chitin biosynthesis. It is both ovicidal and larvicidal. It is very safe for mammals; it concentrates in fat and is slowly released into the blood stream. Sodium polyborate powder kills larvae and eggs by desiccation and is very effective for carpeted areas. It can last for up to 1 year; however, carpets cannot be steam cleaned during this period. Flea control in the outdoor environment involves removal of leaves and mulch from shaded areas, limiting pets access to damp dark areas, and keeping free roaming mammals (cats, dogs, wild small mammals) from living in or around homes and sheds. Pyriproxifen can be sprayed outdoors to control larvae. *Steinernema carpocapsae* are nematodes that eat flea larvae. They come in a powder that is sprinkled over organic debris or in a vial that can be attached to a garden hose and sprayed over the yard.

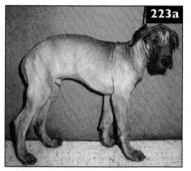
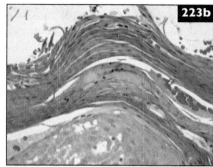

223 A 6-month-old Great Dane puppy was presented for the problem of pruritus (223a). The owner reported that the pruritus had developed gradually over the last 3 months. The puppy's vaccination history was current and the owner administered monthly spot-on flea control. The skin was thickened, erythematous, and scaly. There was no evidence of a bacterial pyoderma (i.e. papules, pustules, epidermal collarettes). The puppy was depressed, febrile, lame, and had lymphadenopathy. Skin scrapings were negative for *Demodex* mites. Skin impression smears revealed large numbers of shed nucleated keratinocytes, but no bacteria or yeast were observed. CBC and serum chemistries were within reported laboratory normal ranges for the dog's age. A FNA of the lymph nodes was compatible with reactive lymph nodes. A skin biopsy was obtained.

i. The key findings of the skin biopsy are shown (223b). The pathologist commented that this finding was diffuse and extended into the hair follicles. What is the diagnosis?

ii. What are the three types of this condition?

iii. What is the treatment?

224 A 2-year-old cat presented for the problem of multiple melanomas of the ears. Close examination of the ears revealed that lesions were limited to the pinna and periauricular skin. A large number of darkly pigmented cysts were present (224). On rupture of the cysts, darkly pigmented, often slightly granular, material exuded out. Once the cyst was ruptured and evacuated the pigmentation disappeared. This is a classic presentation of what condition?

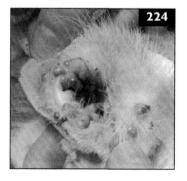

223 i. Zinc-responsive skin disease. The key finding in the skin biopsy is parakeratotic hyperkeratosis. In zinc-responsive skin diseases this abnormality is widespread and since it involves changes in epidermopoiesis, changes extend into the hair follicles, which can be a key diagnostic feature.
ii. Syndrome I occurs in northern or sled dog breeds (e.g. husky, malamute, akita); a genetic defect in zinc absorption is suspected. These dogs present with symmetrical crusted lesions that vary in severity from focal to widespread, with an older age of onset (1–3 years of age). Syndrome II is the result of zinc-deficient diets or diets high in phytates (high plant/grain) and/or calcium. A third syndrome is acrodermatitis, originally described in bull terriers. This rare, inherited autosomal recessive metabolic disease starts at 6–8 weeks of age and is only partially responsive to treatment. Dogs develop crusted skin, growth abnormalities, decreased immune function with chronic diarrhea, and bronchopneumonia. More recently, another breed-related zinc-responsive skin disease has been reported in a litter of Pharaoh hound puppies. Three of five puppies developed severe generalized erythematous and crusted papules with pruritus, marked exfoliation, and erythema of the foot pads. The puppies were inappetent, lethargic, and had retarded growth. Affected puppies were administered intravenous zinc supplementation at 3–4 week intervals to control skin lesions. The dogs were followed for over 2 years; they had stunted growth and enamel hypoplasia of permanent dentition.
iii. Feed a complete and balanced diet and supplement the dog with zinc gluconate, zinc sulfate, or zinc methionine.

224 Feline ceruminous cystomatosis (also known as apocrine hidrocystomas), which can occur in the ears and/or around the eyelids of cats. These masses are referred to as apocrine hidrocystomas, especially when they occur around the eyelids. Lesions are characterized by single to multiple punctate nodules to vesicles in the external ear canal and inner pinna. These lesions are dark blue, brown, or black and can be mistaken for melanocytic or vascular neoplasms. The literature reports this to be an 'old age change' and a disease of older cats, but the lesions are observed frequently in younger cats. These lesions are classic, as rupture of the cysts reveals a black-brown liquid, often with a grainy texture. Diagnosis is clinical; however, biopsy is recommended to rule out melanoma. Skin biopsy reveals cystic glands grouped in clusters. The lesions are best treated via laser surgery or with silver nitrate. Successful treatment using surgical debulking followed by chemical ablation with 20% trichloroacetic acid (used in plastic surgery for cosmetic chemical peels) has been reported.

225 i. What is the difference between cyclosporine and cyclosporine (modified)? How does this difference relate to veterinary medicine?
ii. What diseases has cyclosporine been used to treat?
iii. What are the most common clinical side-effects associated with cyclosporine administration?

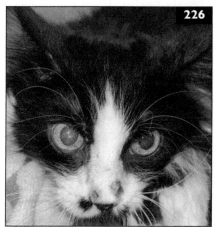

226 A 21-year-old female spayed DSH cat presented for crusting lesions on the haired skin of the bridge of the nose. The cat had numerous other medical illnesses for which she was being managed, but there was no previous history of skin disease. The lesions were not noted to be overly pruritic or uncomfortable. They were confined strictly to the facial location shown (**226**). What are your differential diagnoses for this patient?

225 i. Cyclosporine (modified) is a microemulsion formulation of cyclosporine. The modified form is absorbed more effectively and predictably in small animals, leading to enhanced bioavailability. The non-modified form is influenced by a number of factors, including bile flow, presence of food, and gastrointestinal motility, with regard to systemic absorption.

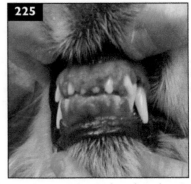

ii. Canine and feline AD, sebaceous adenitis, perianal fistulae, feline eosinophilic skin lesions, feline pseudopelade, sterile nodular panniculitis, CLE, cutaneous reactive histiocytosis, vaccine-induced ischemic dermatopathy, juvenile cellulitis, variable response for PF and PE.

iii. Vomiting, diarrhea, nausea, anorexia, gingival hyperplasia (**225**), hypertrichosis. Diabetes mellitus has been reported rarely in dogs administered cyclosporine for AD; a recent study documented disturbances in glucose metabolism. Blood work abnormalities, including elevations in alkaline phosphatase, alanine aminotransferase, and cholesterol, have been reported by the manufacturer; however, these changes are rarely associated with clinical signs of disease. Other uncommon to rare side-effects in dogs and cats include bacterial infection, bone marrow suppression, hirsutism and excessive shedding, hepatitis, lymphoma and lymphoproliferative disorders, neosporosis, nephropathy, nocardiosis, papillomatosis, seizures, sodium retention, and toxoplasmosis.

226 Include dermatophytosis and demodicosis (although this is a fairly atypical location) because of the concurrent medical illnesses and age of this patient. Other differentials include PF, superficial bacterial pyoderma, drug reaction, foreign body reaction, trauma, mosquito bite hypersensitivity with secondary self-trauma, less likely deep fungal disease (such as cryptococcosis), and neoplasia. In this patient, cytology from under the crust revealed a moderate number of cocci bacteria. Superficial pyoderma was suspected due to previous foreign body reaction/trauma after the cat had inadvertently come into contact with a cactus in the house.

227 A 4-year-old male castrated collie dog was presented for chronic skin lesions on the face, tail, and distal extremities of all four limbs. The lesions consisted of crusting along the bridge of the nose along with scarring alopecia of the muz-

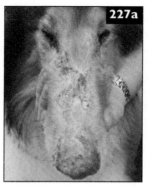

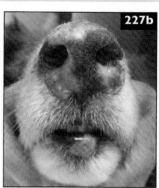

zle and periocular regions (227a), ulceration with crusting, depigmentation and scar formation involving the nasal planum (227b), and scarring alopecia with erythema along the distal aspect of all four limbs (227c). The owner had obtained the dog from a rescue organization and was told that numerous other dogs from the same litter were similarly affected.

i. What is the most likely diagnosis in this patient? What other differential diagnoses would you consider if this dog was a 16-week-old puppy? What if the lesions were present in a different dog breed? What if only the facial lesions were present in this dog?

ii. What other clinical signs may be associated with this condition?

228 In-house cytologic evaluation is an important part of daily dermatologic practice. Collection technique and processing of the sample can impact on the diagnostic sensitivity of disease detection. Accurate interpretation of the cytologic sample can be influenced by where the sample was collected from, how the sample was obtained, and how it was processed prior to evaluation. Otitis externa is a common indication to perform cytology evaluation; the presence or absence of organisms along with what types of organism are seen (e.g. yeast, cocci bacteria, rod-shaped bacteria) will influence the 'next step' diagnostically and therapeutically for many practitioners.

i. What is Diff-Quick® stain?

ii. What options are available with regard to fixation of an ear swab sample?

iii. What options are available for staining ear swabs using a Diff-Quick type of stain?

227 i. The facial lesions are symmetrical, suggesting metabolic or immune-mediated disease (e.g. pemphigus); however, breed and distribution make the most likely diagnosis familial canine dermatomyositis. If the patient originally presented as a young puppy and lesions were inflammatory, pediatric diseases such as demodicosis and dermatophytosis would need to be ruled out prior to diagnostics (i.e. skin biopsy) to confirm a suspicion of juvenile-onset ischemic dermatopathy; this condition presents in very young dogs and without a specific breed association. If the patient was an adult but of a different breed (non-collie or Shetland sheep dog), other causes of ischemic dermatopathy should be considered including vaccination-induced ischemic dermatopathy and idiopathic ischemic dermatopathy. Vaccination-induced ischemic dermatopathy typically has a time course associated with recent vaccination (within 4 months of presentation) and may be localized (at the site of injection) or generalized. If strictly facial lesions are present, lupoid diseases (discoid lupus in particular) would be an important differential diagnosis.
ii. Skeletal muscle atrophy (often most noticeable over the temporal muscles, trunk, and extremities), dermatitis involving scarring alopecia, erythema and crusting over all extremities (head, face, ears, tail, distal limbs, bony prominences), decreased jaw tone, stiff gait, megaesophagus, difficulty breeding, and hyperreflexia have been noted in more severely affected patients.

228 i. A Romanowsky stain variant based on modification of Wright–Giemsa stain. It involves three different solutions into which a dried cytology sample is immersed. The first solution is a fixative reagent, typically with an alcohol base (methanol is most commonly used). The second solution is a xanthene dye (the 'stain'), which stains the sample first eosinophilic. The third solution is a thiazine dye (the 'counterstain'), which stains aspects of the sample basophilic. Intrinsic organism and cellular properties lead to variable appearance of the sample on cytologic evaluation.
ii. Include heat fixing the sample to the slide prior to staining, or proceeding solely with the first Diff-Quick solution after the sample has been allowed to air-dry.
iii. Include using the complete three-step process (fixative, stain, counterstain) or solely the third solution (basophilic counterstain). In a study evaluating the different fixation and staining methods for canine ear swab cytology, it was concluded that heat fixation did not provide appreciable improvement of sample quality compared with non-heat fixed samples. Also, it did not make much difference to cytology interpretation whether the sample was prepared with the three-step method or whether the counterstain alone was used. Inter-observer variation is still a factor in ear swab cytology interpretation, regardless of what fixation and staining methods are utilized.

229 A 5-year-old male castrated Labrador retriever dog presented for an acute history of moderate to severe pruritus and discomfort. The dog had not eaten well that morning and had been lethargic for the past 2 days. On physical examination, the dog was reluctant to move and appeared to be in pain. Diffuse erythema and mild swelling were present periocularly (**229a**) and on the medial aspects of the pinnae. Erythematous macules were noted along with occasional papules and pustules and slightly raised plaques, the latter occasionally appearing 'targetoid', intermixed with normal appearing serpiginous regions (**229b**). Skin surrounding mucous membranes was affected; however, non-haired skin appeared normal. The dog had a rectal temperature of 40.6°C (105.1°F). The owners did not report anything unusual with regard to the dog's history; nothing had changed within the past week and the dog was not receiving any medications.

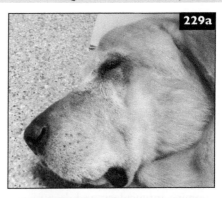

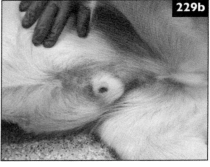

i. Based on the clinical appearance, what are your differential diagnoses for this patient?
ii. Skin biopsy showed diffuse infiltration of the dermis (superficial and deep) with large numbers of neutrophils, often clustering along the hair follicles. Occasional neutrophilic infiltration crossed into the epidermis, forming small intraepidermal pustules. Severe edema was present throughout the dermis. Based on this information, what additional diagnostics are indicated?
iii. CBC showed marked peripheral neutrophilia. Provided your additional diagnostics from Qii are negative, what is your diagnosis?

230 A i. What is the pathogenesis of the dermatomyositis diagnosed in case **227**?
ii. What are the treatment options?

229 i. EM, bacterial pyoderma (superficial and/or deep), fungal infection (histoplasmosis, cryptococcosis, sporotrichosis), neoplasia (cutaneous lymphoma, mast cell tumor), canine eosinophilic dermatitis (Wells syndrome), sterile neutrophilic dermatitis (Sweet's syndrome), toxic shock syndrome, post-grooming furunculosis, sterile erythroderma (typically seen only in miniature schnauzer dogs).

ii. CBC and serum biochemistries to screen for peripheral leukocyte abnormalities and determine whether there is a known source of the fever; special stains (GMS, PAS, Fite's) to assess the presence of infectious organisms on skin biopsy samples; bacterial and fungal cultures.

iii. Sterile neutrophilic dermatitis or Sweet's syndrome. This disease may take a form similar to EM in which macules, small papules, pustules, and slightly raised plaques predominate, or more distinct nodular lesions may be present. Post-grooming furunculosis and deep pyoderma must be ruled out. Sweet's syndrome in dogs tends to mimic the disease in people; sterile neutrophilic infiltration of the skin is reported along with peripheral neutrophilia, and patients are often febrile. Other body organs may also be infiltrated. Strictly, sterile neutrophilic infiltration of the dermis and epidermis in the absence of extracutaneous signs may also occur.

230 i. Familial dermatomyositis is a congenital/hereditary disease most commonly reported in collies and Shetland sheep dogs and their crosses. Other breeds may show similar clinical signs, but the underlying cause (i.e. genetics) is different. The condition develops due to ischemic injury to the skin and skeletal muscles. The disease varies in severity. Previous work done with collies has documented an autosomal dominant inheritance with incomplete penetrance. In Shetland sheep dogs, a linkage to chromosome 35 has been documented in disease development. Additional studies have identified numerous gene transcripts associated with immune function, but have not determined specific autoantibodies or genetic defects associated with familial dermatomyositis in Shetland sheep dogs.

ii. There is no cure for familial canine dermatomyositis because this is a genetic disease. Pentoxifylline has been shown to be effective in many patients. Supplementation with essential fatty acids and vitamin E may also be beneficial. For either drug, it can take up to 3 months before any noticeable benefit is seen. In more severe cases, prednisone is administered and then tapered to control flares of the disease; long-term administration will worsen muscle atrophy. Management should also include bathing to minimize crust formation and decrease the frequency of secondary bacterial pyoderma, which commonly develops.

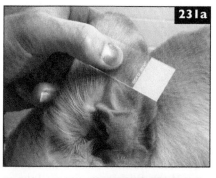

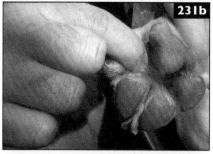

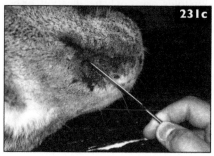

231 Examination of skin cytology is an important diagnostic test. Skin cytology can be collected using a glass microscope slide (**231a**), clear acetate tape preparation (**231b**), or by scraping debris from under nails or skin folds with a skin-scraping spatula (**231c**). Briefly describe how optimum specimens are obtained using each of these three techniques.

232 Fleas can transmit a variety of infectious diseases. List at least three infectious diseases that are transmitted by fleas.

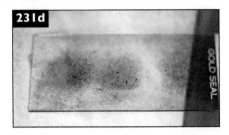

231

- Glass microscope slide. Always use a new glass microscope slide. Place the slide directly over the target area and then place a thumb over the site and gently press once only to avoid too thick a specimen. Take multiple samplings on the same slide using different sites (**231d**). Samples from intact pustules are obtained by gently rupturing the pustule with a sterile needle. Samples from crusted lesions are obtained by lifting the crust and getting the sample from beneath. The specimen must be allowed to dry completely before and after staining. Adequately sampled specimens should show a clear 'fingerprint' (**231d**).

- Acetate tape. Press clear acetate tape over the target site, skip the 'fixative step' to avoid fogging tape, allow the specimen to dry before mounting, and mount over a drop of immersion oil.

- Scraping technique. A skin-scraping spatula is used to collect material from beneath nail beds, skin folds, areas of lichenification, or beneath crusts. Material collected from these sites is spread over the surface of a glass microscope slide before staining. This technique is especially useful for looking for yeast beneath nail folds.

232 The most severe infection spread by fleas is *Yersina pestis*. In addition, they can spread *Rickettsia typhi* (murine typhus, which is a worldwide zoonosis), *R. prowazekii* (present in the USA and known as rural endemic typhus), *R. felis* (flea-borne spotted fever), *Bartonella henselae* (cat scratch fever), *Bartonella quintana* (trench fever; the primary host is the human louse but fleas can also spread this disease). Fleas also act as hosts for the helminth parasites *Dipylidium caninum* (tapeworms) and *Hymenolepis diminuta*.

233 A 7-year-old male castrated yellow Labrador retriever dog presented for acute severe pruritus and appearance of a large skin lesion (233). The owners had noted the dog shaking his head a bit more frequently for the past week. However, the lesion was not present prior to the owners going to bed the night before presentation. No other lesions were noted on examination.

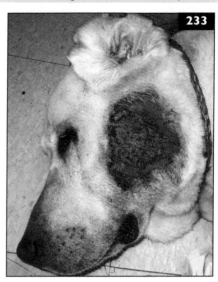

i. What are the differential diagnoses for this patient based on clinical appearance?
ii. Of the differential diagnoses, which is most likely given the history?
iii. What diagnostic tests do you recommend for this patient?
iv. With regard to 'hot spots', what is the classification of this lesion?
v. What are the treatment options?

234 A 6-month-old kitten was presented for evaluation of non-responsive unilateral otitis externa. Initial ear swab cytology revealed neutrophils, cocci, and yeast. Initial treatment for the microbial overgrowth did not resolve the otitis. Examination of the ear revealed proliferative, erythematous necrotic tissue covering the proximal pinna and vertical ear canal (234). The ear was pruritic and painful. Skin biopsy revealed sharp demarcation between normal and abnormal tissue. There were scattered apoptotic appearing keratinocytes within severely hyperplastic epithelium. The abnormalities also affected hair

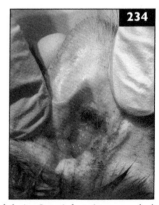

follicles, which were dilated and filled with necrotic debris. Special stains revealed CD3+ T cells and caspase-3-stained keratinocytes, consistent with keratinocyte apoptosis by epidermal infiltrating T cells. What is the most likely diagnosis, and how is this treated?

233 i. Pyotraumatic dermatitis, demodicosis, dermatophytosis, superficial pyoderma, deep pyoderma, neoplasia (mast cell tumor, apocrine gland tumor, cutaneous metastasis), drug eruption.
ii. Pyotraumatic dermatitis because of the acute onset of the lesion.
iii. Deep skin scraping, otoscopic examination, ear swab cytology to look for evidence of otitis externa. Culture and susceptibility may be needed based on the dog's previous antibiotic exposure.
iv. 'Hot spot' (pyotraumatic dermatitis, acute moist dermatitis) is a common example of acute superficial bacterial pyoderma. Histologically, there are two presentations: superficial and deep pyoderma.
v. The hair coat needs to clipped and then cleansed with an antimicrobial topical shampoo or scrub. The dog may need to be sedated as these lesions can be severely pruritic and/or painful. These lesions are best treated with focal antimicrobial therapy. Previous studies have advocated the use of systemic antibiotics; this should be considered when evidence of spreading superficial pyoderma is also present. With the increasing prevalence of resistant organisms and the overriding focus on judicious antibiotic use, topical control alone may be sufficient in many cases. Some animals may also require the addition of mechanical restraints (e.g. Elizabethan collar, socks, shirts) to prevent scratching and further trauma. Addressing the underlying cause of the pruritus/pain is also recommended to help prevent further pyotraumatic dermatitis lesions from developing.

234 Proliferative and necrotizing otitis. This is a uniquely and visually distinctive ear lesion. Lesions can occur in kittens between 2 and 6 months of age and may or may not spontaneously regress by 12–24 months of age. The lesions may respond to glucocorticoids or to tacrolimus; however, effective treatment is not always possible. This disease is considered rare, but it may simply be unrecognized.

235 Four 6-mm punch biopsies from the skin of the lateral trunk of a 6-year-old neutered male standard poodle dog with hair coat abnormalities (**235**) have been submitted for dermatopathologic examination.

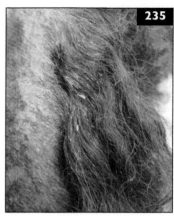

Histological report: the epidermis is normal thickness and there is marked diffuse ortho-keratosis and follicular keratosis. Sebaceous glands are diffusely absent. Adjacent to a few follicles, at the level of the isthmus, are tiny aggregates of lymphocytes, mast cells, and macrophages. Hair follicles have a stretched out appearance and occasional follicles have an irregular outline and contain an irregular dystrophic hair shaft. In one biopsy, several follicles are atrophic and are in non-haired telogen.

Morphological diagnosis: diffuse sebaceous gland atrophy, with focal minimal parafolliculitis, marked orthokeratosis, follicular keratosis, and multifocal hair follicle atrophy.

i. What is the diagnosis based on the histopathologic description?
ii. Which breeds of dog are predisposed to this disease?
iii. What is the suspected mode of inheritance of this disease in standard poodle dogs?
iv. What other species has it been reported to affect?

236 A 4-year-old cat presented for the complaint of 'bumps'. Palpation of the skin followed by clipping of the hair coat revealed multiple, firm nodules on the lateral aspect of the thigh (**236**). The lesions were non-painful when manipulated. The medical record indicated that the last time the cat was examined was at the age of 1 year when it was vaccinated. When asked about the onset of the masses, the owner reported that they occurred suddenly and have rapidly developed over the last 2 weeks. The cat is otherwise healthy.

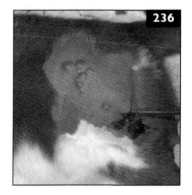

i. What are possible differential diagnoses?
ii. What is the 3-2-1 rule?
iii. The skin biopsy is compatible with a sarcoma. What is the treatment?

235 i. Sebaceous adenitis (SA) given the relative absence of sebaceous glands and aggregates of inflammation where these glands are normally found.
ii. Standard poodle, vizsla, samoyed, akita, and English springer spaniel dog breeds are believed to be predisposed. Dachshunds, Belgian sheepdogs, and Havanese breed dogs may be at increased risk for SA.
iii. An autosomal recessive mode of inheritance is strongly suspected.
iv. SA has been reported in dogs, cats, rabbits, horses, and humans.

236 i. The dermatologic problem is 'tumor' and there are three major causes: infections, granulomas (sterile inflammatory), and neoplasia. The most common infection in the cat is an abscess, but clinically these lesions are not compatible with abscesses. Subcutaneous infections with opportunistic fungi can appear similarly; however, lesions are usually slow to develop. Granulomatous reactions in cats are uncommon. They can occur as a result of tick or flea bites, but these are usually smaller in size and slower to develop. Pansteatitis as a result of poor diet can occur, but these lesions are typically painful. The most likely cause is subcutaneous skin tumor; injection-site sarcoma is most likely.
ii. The Vaccine Associated Feline Sarcoma Task Force (VAFSTF) recommends for every mass that (a) persists for >3 months after injection, (b) becomes larger than 2 cm, and/or (c) increases in size 1 month after injection should be biopsied (3-2-1 rule). If fibrosarcoma is suspected, an incisional biopsy specimen is recommended (not a Tru-cut); the tumor can be heterogenous and misdiagnosed as a granuloma from small tissue samples.
iii. The mainstay of treatment is wide surgical excision with a goal of a 3–5 cm macroscopic margin of healthy tissue and at least one fascial plane beneath the tumor. Radical surgery greatly affects recurrence rate. Radiation therapy with or without chemotherapy can follow. Cats with the best prognosis are those that undergo aggressive surgery and are treated with multiple modalities.

237 Sebaceous adenitis (SA) is an inflammatory skin disease in which sebaceous glands are specifically targeted, as shown by the histopathology report in case **235**.

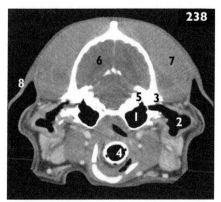

i. How is the histopathologic pattern different in short-coated breeds of dogs (**237a**) compared with standard poodle dogs?

ii. List other diseases whose cellular infiltrate might incidentally surround, disrupt, or destroy sebaceous glands as seen histopathologically.

iii. Describe what this dog's skin might look like given the disease process.

238 A CT scan is frequently incorporated into the diagnostics for a dog or cat with chronic and/or recurrent ear disease, particularly when middle ear involvement is suspected. In general, the sensitivity and specificity of CT are much higher than those of plain film radiography in cases of moderate to severe otitis. CT scans may also be incorporated with virtual otoscopy to provide a more accurate image in a non-invasive setting.

i. Is this CT scan (**238**) from a dog or a cat?

ii. Identify the labeled structures on the scan.

237 i. Short-coated dogs affected by SA, such as the vizsla, usually have large discrete periadnexal nodules composed of granulomatous to pyogranulomatous inflammation centered where there should normally be sebaceous glands (follicular isthmus). Inflammation at the isthmus level tends to be less prominent in standard poodles, especially during the late stages of disease.

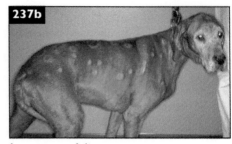

ii. Demodicosis, dermatophytosis, leishmaniosis, reactive histiocytosis, sterile granuloma/pyogranuloma syndrome, uveodermatologic syndrome, pseudopelade, exfoliative cutaneous lupus erythematosus of the German shorthaired pointer, epitheliotropic lymphoma. Other histopathologic findings and patient signalment help discriminate these diseases from SA; however, clinical differentiation might be required in select cases.

iii. Initially, standard poodle dogs with SA develop with excessive and adherent white surface scale that is not overtly pruritic. Follicular seborrhea, manifested comedones, and fronds of keratinous material protruding from follicular ostia/openings and entrapping exiting hair shafts (**237b**) are also common findings. As the disease progresses a dull, dry, brittle coat with broken hairs that is multifocal to generalized is seen. Loss of the normal 'crimp' to the hair denotes an additional change in coat quality. These lesions first arise on the muzzle, head, pinnae, neck, and dorsolateral trunk before extending to other body areas. Papules, pustules, crusts, and pruritus may be a feature when bacterial folliculitis is present.

238 i. Dog. The presence of pendulous pinnae on the scan identifies the animal as a dog. Cats have a prominent bony shelf separating the tympanic bulla into two distinct compartments.

ii. 1 = tympanic bulla; 2 = external ear canal (near the level of the vertical and horizontal canal); 3 = tympanic membrane; 4 = trachea (outlined by radiopaque endotracheal tube); 5 = inner ear ossicles; 6 = brain; 7 = temporal muscles; 8 = pinna.

239 A 5-year-old female spayed Labrador retriever dog was evaluated for lethargy, anorexia, and erythematous skin lesions. At presentation, the dog was febrile (40.7°C [105°F]) with dull mentation. When the hair coat was clipped, well-circumscribed erythematous lesions were present over the entire body (**239**). There were no lesions found on the mucous membranes. Four days prior to the

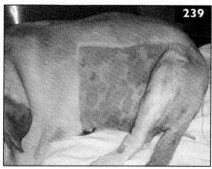

development of the recent clinical signs, the dog chewed on bones from a turkey carcass for several hours until the owners discarded the remains.

i. Based on the patient's history and physical examination, what differentials should be considered?

ii. What diagnostic tests are indicated in this patient?

iii. Blood cultures are positive and the laboratory's preliminary findings identify a small gram-positive anaerobic rod. Considering the history and clinical signs, what is the most likely diagnosis, and what other comorbidities should be evaluated in this patient?

iv. Your diagnosis is confirmed and a skin biopsy is needed. What would you expect to find on skin biopsy?

v. What is the best treatment?

240 These lesions developed over a 1-month period (**240**). The owners reported that the dog vocalized one evening and within hours there was marked swelling of the face. Within days, a non-healing wound developed. Skin biopsy of the tissue revealed necrosis and no etiological agents. Bacterial culture of the wound and of tissue did not isolate any bacteria.

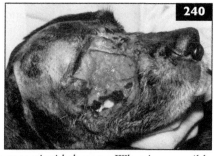

The lesions have progressed in spite of glucocorticoid therapy. What is a possible inciting cause?

239 i. Vasculitis, thrombocytopenia/thrombopathia, coagulopathy, cutaneous drug eruption.

ii. CBC, serum chemistry panel, skin biopsy, blood culture, and urine culture should be considered if the dog is not in a hypercoagulable state.

iii. *Erysipelothrix rhusiopathiae*, which is the causative agent of diamond skin disease in pigs. *Erysipelothrix* organisms are epitheliotropic and damage endothelial cell barriers, leading to local cellulitis with edema. Wild birds and mammals can also harbor *E. rhusiopathiae*, and thus are potential reservoirs of the microorganism. It is likely that this patient acquired the bacteria while she was chewing on a turkey carcass 4 days prior to the development of clinical signs. During chewing, damage to the oral mucosa likely occurred, allowing translocation of bacteria from the carrion.

iv. *E. rhusiopathiae* infection typically results in cellulitis with marked edema in the upper and mid dermis, vascular dilatation, and neutrophilic, lymphocytic, and eosinophilic inflammatory infiltrate in the upper and mid dermis.

v. Antibiotic therapy should be guided by results of blood and urine culture susceptibility findings. If empiric antibiotic therapy is needed while cultures are pending, or if cultures were not obtained, previous reports show that *E. rhusiopathiae* is highly susceptible to penicillins and cephalosporins; these drugs should be considered first-line therapy.

240 Envenomation by an insect or snake secreting a necrotizing toxin was suspected to be the inciting cause after infectious agents were ruled out. The vocalization was most likely the bite and the swelling the initial reaction. The progressive necrosis suggests a dermonecrotic toxin. There are two spiders (recluse spider and sixed-eyed sand spider) that are known to secrete a dermonecrotic agent called sphingomyelinase D. Initial bites often start as a 'halo' with a vesicle and progress to a black necrotic area. Lesions can become very large; in some cases systemic signs can occur within 24–72 hours and include hemolysis, hematuria, fever, and arthralgia.

241 A 4-year-old female spayed golden retriever dog presented for acute onset of lameness in all four feet. The dog had been out running, swimming, and hiking over the weekend; the weather had been quite warm at the time. The owner noted that over the next 2 days the dog seemed to be limping, which progressed to shifting limb lameness and not wanting to walk, especially on hard and uneven surfaces. The dog had

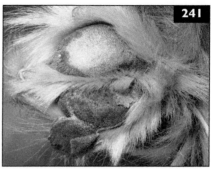

also been licking its paws more frequently, paying equal attention to the front and rear paws. The dog was not receiving any medication other than topical flea and heartworm prevention once monthly year round. She was otherwise healthy with no previous dermatologic abnormalities. On physical examination, all four paws had a similar appearance (241) with primarily the paw pads affected; only mild interdigital erythema was noted on the haired skin. No other lesions were noted on the dog; all mucous membranes appeared normal.

i. What are the differential diagnoses for the condition noted?
ii. Given the history and clinical appearance, what is the most likely diagnosis?
iii. What is the proposed mechanism for the disease in dogs?

242 A 3-year-old Labrador retriever dog was presented for the problem of year-round pruritus. The dog was receiving year-round flea and tick control, skin scrapings were negative, and contagious mites had been ruled out via a response to treatment trial using ivermectin. At the time of initial presentation, the dog had clinical signs consistent with bacterial pyoderma and yeast overgrowth was confirmed via skin cytology. Culture and sensitivity isolated an SIG isolate susceptible to cephalexin. After 30 days of cephalexin and oral ketoconazole, the pruritus persisted despite resolution of clinical lesions associated with microbial overgrowth. At this point the differential diagnoses were narrowed to food allergy and/or canine AD. The owner completed a home-cooked food elimination trial using kangaroo meat, lentils, and potatoes for 8 weeks. There was no change in pruritus during the diet or during the re-introduction of the previous food. At this point the working diagnosis was AD and an IDT was performed. Based on identification of several positive reactions, the owner was given the options of sole medical therapy (i.e. cyclosporine) or immunotherapy; the owner elected immunotherapy. What do you need to consider when selecting allergens for immunotherapy?

241 i. PF (confined to the paw pads), zinc-responsive skin disease, superficial necrolytic dermatitis, split paw-pad syndrome, generic dog food dermatosis, drug eruption.
ii. Split paw-pad syndrome.
iii. The exact etiology is unknown; however, an anatomic defect in paw-pad cornification is suspected. The disease has a characteristic clinical appearance in which the paw pad becomes split and then peels off much of the superficial layer, leaving a defect in the pad and exposed lower epidermal layers. The adjacent haired skin is generally unaffected. Dogs can heal normally or with irregular, lumpy keratinized pads; the latter can cause chronic inflammatory changes. Trauma and exposure to moisture may precipitate an episode of split paw-pad syndrome. Self-trauma may exacerbate lesions; dogs will frequently pull off torn, ripped fragments with their teeth.

242 IDT can identify reactions to all major allergen groups (trees, grasses, weeds, indoor allergens). It is not possible or practical to include all allergens into the ASIT prescription. Although the exact amount of allergen necessary to stimulate an appropriate immunologic response is not known, most allergen prescriptions contain 10–12 allergens. Flea bite hypersensitivity is best managed with flea control rather than immunotherapy. Mold allergy cannot be discounted and there may be regional variations. Management of mold allergy can often be addressed via avoidance and environmental changes in addition to ASIT. Currently, the key steps are to decrease humidity in the home, instruct clients not to house the dog in areas typically high in molds (laundry rooms, bathrooms, basements, cellars), and improve air filtration via furnace filters. Look for allergens that can be managed strictly by avoidance (e.g. wool, feathers). Look for results that do not match the exposure history. For example, if the dog has strong reactions to grasses, but is not pruritic during the grass season, these allergens are less important to include in the allergy prescription. Finally, review the laboratory results for cross-reactivity between plant families. Selection of one or a few allergens from each botanical group that showed positive reactions may suffice.

243 A 6-month-old male castrated mixed-breed dog presents for multifocal areas of partial alopecia. The owners first noted a spot of hair missing on the top of the head; however, three other areas have developed on the dog's face within the past week. You perform a deep skin scraping and identify *Demodex canis*.
i. Depending on the temperament of your patient as well as lesion location, collecting a diagnostic sample with a deep skin scraping can at times be difficult. What tools may be used for collecting a deep skin scraping?
ii. Other than deep skin scrapings, by what other methods can demodicosis be diagnosed? Which methods tend to be most accurate?
iii. *D. canis* is known to be a 'normal' inhabitant of the canine skin. If *Demodex* mites are found by one of the diagnostic methods discussed, how likely are they to be pathogenic as opposed to 'normal'?

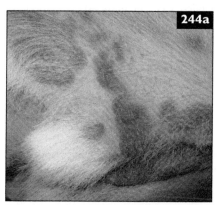

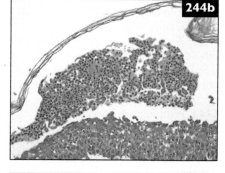

244 A 5-year-old mixed-breed dog was presented for pustular lesions on the face, ears, paw pads, and ventrum (**244a**). Skin biopsy findings revealed multifocal subcorneal intact (**244b**) and non-intact (**244c**) pustules with large numbers of acantholytic cells.
i. What is the most likely diagnosis in this case?
ii. What other differential diagnoses should be considered taking into consideration the biopsy findings?
iii. In cases of pustular dermatitis, how should skin biopsies be collected?

243 i. Shown in 243. A scalpel blade is commonly used for collecting samples by means of deep skin scraping. In mobile patients or for areas of sensitive skin (e.g. periocular), laceration is possible. This is true for both the patient and the veterinarian; this technique is considered to be a 'high-risk factor' for exposure to human blood in the work place. A laboratory spatula with a rounded tip is preferred; the tip is scraped along the direction of hair growth with applied pressure to obtain capillary 'oozing'. This is the authors' preferred method.

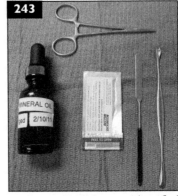

ii. Exudative cytology, hair plucking, biopsy. Exudative cytology is beneficial when deep pyoderma is present; mites are identified by cytologic examination of debris. Hair plucking is useful for sampling areas that are difficult to scrape (e.g. periocular tissue, muzzle); mites are present near the base of hair shafts. Skin biopsy is recommended when demodicosis is suspected, but cannot be found using less invasive tests.

iii. In healthy dogs, the prevalence of mites found should not exceed a threshold of 5.4% of the population. If *Demodex* mites are found on skin scraping, they should be considered important; repeated skin scrapings to confirm their presence is indicated if the patient is 'not clinical' for skin disease to assure the finding was not aberrant.

244 i. Pemphigus foliaceus.

ii. Occasionally, acantholytic cells can be observed in cases of dermatophytosis. Acantholytic cells can be seen in cases of severe deep pyoderma or chronic pyoderma. Special stains and fungal culture can be used to rule out dermatophytosis. To rule out the possibility of the pustular lesions with acantholytic cells being due to a chronic pyoderma, intact pustules should be collected and submitted for histologic examination.

iii. They should be collected preferentially from areas with intact and early developing pustules. If large pustules are present, a punch biopsy should be avoided, because the rotation of the punch could result in disruption of the lesions. In this case, and in cases of vesicular dermatitis, an excisional biopsy is preferred. Chronic lesions with superficial crusts should also be submitted, preferentially intact. If crusts slough from the adjacent skin, these should also be submitted for histologic examination. Even though intact pustules are preferred, superficial crusts can frequently assist in diagnosing PF.

245 A 2-year-old female spayed golden retriever dog was referred for the problem of recurrent *Pseudomonas* bacterial pyoderma. Past pertinent history revealed that the dog was diagnosed as having 'allergies' at approximately 6 months of age. The owners elected medical management and were applying an unknown topical product to the skin. At the time of presentation the dog had extensive hair loss, self-trauma and raised erythematous papules and plaques on the dorsum, neck, trunk, and vulvar area (245a). The lesions were pruritic and exudative at the margins. Culture confirmed the bacteria as SIG (heavy growth) and *Pseudomonas* spp. (scant growth).

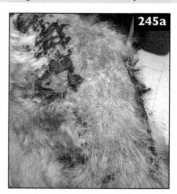

i. How do you interpret the *Pseudomonas* isolation?

ii. *Pseudomonas* pyoderma has been reported in dogs. What are the clinical signs?

iii. A skin biopsy of the plaques was obtained and the results are shown (245b). What is the diagnosis, and what are possible causes of this disease?

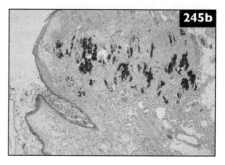

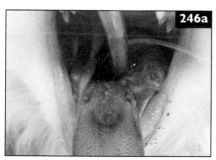

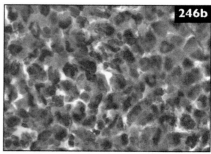

246 The oral cavity of a 6-year-old orange tabby cat is shown (246a). Note the oral lesions in the mouth. The owner presented the cat for examination because of excessive drooling, lack of appetite, and odor.

i. What are the most likely differential diagnoses?

ii. Touch preparation cytology of the cut edge of a biopsy specimen revealed these cells (246b). What additional differential diagnosis can be considered?

245 i. It represents overgrowth of a transient organism.

ii. In a retrospective study, seven out of twenty dogs with *Pseudomonas* pyoderma presented with deep pyoderma characterized by sudden onset of acute dorsal truncal pain. Lesions consisted of erythematous papules, hemorrhagic bullae, ulcers, and hemorrhagic crusts. The other dogs presented with more gradual onset of lesions and histories of prior skin disease and multidrug antibiotic administration. In these dogs, bacteria were not always noted on cytology; diagnosis was made via culture.

iii. Calcinosis cutis (CC). There is extensive replacement of the dermal collagen by dark-staining material (dystrophic mineralization). The most common cause is hypercortisolemia from either endogenous (adrenal gland disease) or exogenous (glucocorticoid administration) sources. CC can occur via percutaneous penetration of calcium chloride or calcium-containing bone meal from landscaping materials, most commonly observed in animals sleeping on supply bags. CC can occur as a complication of intravenous or subcutaneous calcium chloride or calcium gluconate therapy for hypoparathyroidism. Idiopathic CC has been seen in puppies with severe illness. Calcinosis circumscripta is another condition in which dystrophic mineralization of collagen occurs. In this disease, there is focal deposition of mineral salts in a tumor-like presentation. The etiology is unknown, but trauma is considered likely, as lesions are found on pressure points or sites of previous trauma; it has also been found in the oral cavity with no easy explanation.

246 i. Include SCC, fibrosarcoma, and melanoma.

ii. This slide shows a full field of intense eosinophilic infiltrate. An additional differential diagnosis to consider is an eosinophilic inflammatory lesion. The diagnosis in this case was an eosinophilic granuloma complex-like lesion. The cat received three injections of methylprednisolone acetate; the lesion resolved and did not recur.

References

2

Blondeau JM (2009) New concepts in antimicrobial susceptibility testing: the mutant prevention concentration and mutant selection window approach. *Vet Dermatol* 20:383–396.

3

Angles JM, Famula TR, Pedersen NC (2005) Uveodermatologic (VKH-like) syndrome in American Akita dogs is associated with an increased frequency of DQA1*00201. *Tissue Antigens* 66:656–665.

Blackwood SE, Barrie KP, Plummer CE et al. (2011) Uveodermatologic syndrome in a rat terrier. *J Am Anim Hosp Assoc* 47:e56–63.

Laus JL, Sousa MG, Cabral VP et al. (2004) Uveodermatologic syndrome in a Brazilian Fila dog. *Vet Ophthalmol* 7:193–196.

Pye CC (2009) Uveodermatologic syndrome in an Akita. *Can Vet J* 50:861–864.

6

Bauer JE (2011) Therapeutic use of fish oils in companion animals. *J Am Vet Med Assoc* 239:1441–1451.

Kirby NA, Hester SL, Bauer JE (2007) Dietary fats and the skin and coat of dogs. *J Am Vet Med Assoc* 230:1641–1644.

Mueller RS, Rosychuk RA, Jonas LD (2003) A retrospective study regarding the treatment of lupoid onychodystrophy in 30 dogs and literature review. *J Am Anim Hosp Assoc* 39:139–150.

Park HJ, Park JS, Hayek MG et al. (2011) Dietary fish oil and flaxseed oil suppress inflammation and immunity in cats. *Vet Immunol Immunopathol* 141:301–306.

Tretter S, Mueller RS (2011) The influence of topical unsaturated fatty acids and essential oils on normal and atopic dogs. *J Am Anim Hosp Assoc* 47:236–240.

8

Blondeau JM (2009) New concepts in antimicrobial susceptibility testing: the mutant prevention concentration and mutant selection window approach. *Vet Dermatol* 20:383–396.

Dong Y, Zhao, X, Domagala J et al. (1999) Effect of fluoroquinolone concentration on selection of resistant mutants of *Mycobacterium bovis* BCG and *Staphylococcus aureus*. *Antimicrob Agents Chemother* 43:1756–1758.

Drlica K, Zhao X (2007) The mutant selection window hypothesis updated. *Clin Infect Dis* 44:681–688.

9

Anders BB, Hoelzler MG, Scavelli TD et al. (2008) Analysis of auditory and neurologic effects associated with ventral bulla osteotomy for removal of inflammatory polyps or nasopharyngeal masses in cats. *J Am Vet Med Assoc* 233:580–585.

11

Cohn LA, Kerl ME, Lenox CE et al. (2007) Response of healthy dogs to infusions of human serum albumin. *Am J Vet Res* 68:657–663.

Prussin C, Metcalfe DD (2003) IgE, mast cells, basophils, and eosinophils. *J Allergy Clin Immunol* 111:S486–494.

12

Dryden MW, Gaafar SM (1991) Blood consumption by the cat flea, *Ctenocephalides felis* (Siphonaptera: Pulicidae). *J Med Entomol* 28:394–400.

13

Bond R, Curtis CF, Ferguson EA et al. (2000) An idiopathic facial dermatitis of Persian cats. *Vet Dermatol* 11:35–41.

Chung TH, Ryu MH, Kim DY et al. (2009) Topical tacrolimus (FK506) for the treatment of feline idiopathic facial dermatitis. *Aust Vet J* 87:417–420.

References

17

Heinrich NA, McKeever PJ, Eisenschenk MC (2011) Adverse events in 50 cats with allergic dermatitis receiving ciclosporin. *Vet Dermatol* 22:511–520.

Hobi S, Linek M, Marignac G *et al.* (2011) Clinical characteristics and causes of pruritus in cats: a multicentre study on feline hypersensitivity-associated dermatoses. *Vet Dermatol* 22:406–413.

18

Correia TR, Scott FB, Verocai GG *et al.* (2010) Larvicidal efficacy of nitenpyram on the treatment of myiasis caused by *Cochliomyia hominivorax* (Diptera: Calliphoridae) in dogs. *Vet Parasitol* 173:169–172.

Hovda LR, Hoser SB (2002) Toxicology of newer pesticides for use in dogs and cats. *Vet Clin North Am Small Anim Pract* 32:455–467.

19

Scott DW (1987) Sterile eosinophilic pustulosis in dog and man: comparative aspects. *J Am Acad Dermatol* 16:1022–1026.

20

Cunliffe WJ, Holland DB, Jeremy A (2004) Comedone formation: etiology, clinical presentation, and treatment. *Clin Dermatol* 22:367–374.

Jazic E, Coyner K, Loeffler D (2006) An evaluation of the clinical, cytological, infectious and histopathological features of feline acne. *Vet Dermatol* 17:134–140.

21

Schuepbach RA, Feistritzer C, Fernández JA *et al.* (2009) Protection of vascular barrier integrity by activated protein C in murine models depends on protease-activated receptor-1. *Thromb Haemostasis* 101:724–733.

Tressel SL, Kaneider NC, Kasuda S *et al.* (2011) A matrix metalloprotease-PAR1 system regulates vascular integrity, systemic inflammation and death in sepsis. *EMBO Mol Med* 3:370–384.

Yilmaz Z, Eralp O, Ilcol YO (2008) Evaluation of platelet count and its association with plateletcrit, mean platelet volume, and platelet size distribution width in a canine model of endotoxemia. *Vet Clin Pathol* 37:159–163.

22

Bitam I, Dittmar K, Parola P *et al.* (2010) Fleas and flea-borne diseases: review. *Int J Infect Dis* 14:e667–e676.

23

DeBay MC (2010) Primary immunodeficiences of dogs and cats. *Vet Clin North Am Small Anim Pract* 40:425–438.

Prieur DJ, Collier LL (1981) Inheritance of the Chediak–Higashi syndrome in cats. *J Hered* 72:175–177.

24

Veir JK, Lappin MR (2010) Molecular diagnostic assays for infectious diseases in cats. *Vet Clin North Am Small Anim Pract* 40:1189–1200.

25

Veir JK, Lappin MR (2010) Molecular diagnostic assays for infectious diseases in cats. *Vet Clin North Am Small Anim Pract* 40:1189–1200.

27

DeBoer and Hillier (2010) unpublished data.

28

Bryden SL, White SD, Dunston SM *et al.* (2005) Clinical, histological and immunological characteristics of exfoliative cutaneous lupus erythematosus in 25 German short-haired pointers. *Vet Dermatol* 16:239–252.

Mauldin EA, Morris DO, Brown DC (2010) Exfoliative cutaneous lupus erythematosus in German short-haired pointer dogs: disease development, progression and evaluation of three immunomodulatory drugs (ciclosporin, hydroxychloroquine, and adalimumab) in a controlled environment. *Vet Dermatol* **21**:373–382.

Vroom MW, Theaker MJ, Rest J et al. (1995) Lupoid dermatosis in five German short-haired pointers. *Vet Dermatol* **6**:93–98.

Want P, Zangerl B, Werner P et al. (2010) Familial cutaneous lupus erythematosus (CLE) in the German shorthaired pointer maps to CFA18, a canine orthologue to human CLE. *Immunogenetics* **63**:197–207.

32

Kano R, Okabayashi K, Nakamura Y et al. (2006) Systemic treatment of sterile panniculitis with tacrolimus and prednisolone in dogs. *J Vet Med Sci* **68**:95–96.

Nghiem P, Pearson G, Langley RG (2002) Tacrolimus and pimecrolimus: from clever prokaryotes to inhibiting calcineurin and treating atopic dermatitis. *J Am Acad Dermatol* **46**:228–241.

Stanley BJ, Hauptman JG (2009) Long-term prospective evaluation of topically applied 0.1% tacrolimus ointment for treatment of perianal sinuses in dogs. *J Am Vet Med Assoc* **235**:397–404.

33

Barros MB, Schubach AO, Valle AC et al. (2004) Cat transmitted sporotrichosis epidemic in Rio de Janeiro, Brazil: description of a series of cases. *Clin Infect Dis* **38**:529–539.

Fernandes GF, Lopes-Bezerra LM, Bernardes-Engemann AR et al. (2011) Serodiagnosis of sporotrichosis infection in cats by enzyme-linked immunosorbent assay using a specific antigen, SsCBF, and crude exoantigens. *Vet Microbiol* **147**:445–449.

Pereira SA, Menezes RC, Gremiao ID et al. (2011) Sensitivity of cytological examination in the diagnosis of feline sporotrichosis. *J Feline Med Surg* **13**:220–223.

Pereira SA, Passos SRL, Silva JN et al. (2010) Response to azolic antifungal agents for treating sporotrichosis. *Vet Rec* **166**:290–294.

Schubach TM, Schubach Ade O, Cuzzi-Maya T et al. (2004) Evaluation of an epidemic of sporotrichosis in cats: 347 cases (1998–2001). *J Am Vet Med Assoc* **2249**:1623–1629.

34

Guardabassi L, Loeber ME, Jacobson A (2004) Transmission of multiple antimicrobial-resistant *Staphylococcus intermedius* between dogs affected by deep pyoderma and their owners. *Vet Microbiol* **98**:23–27.

Mahoudeau I, Delabranche X, Prevost G et al. (1997) Frequency of isolation of *Staphylococcus intermedius* from humans. *J Clin Microbiol* **35**:2153–2154.

Morris DO, Boston RC, O'Shea K et al. (2010) The prevalence of carriage of meticillin-resistant staphylococci by veterinary dermatology practice staff and their respective pets. *Vet Dermatol* **21**:400–407.

35

Greene CE (2012) *Infectious Diseases of the Dog and Cat*, 4th edn. Saunders–Elsevier, St. Louis.

Persico P, Roccabianca R, Corona A et al. (2011) Detection of feline herpes virus 1 via polymerase chain reaction and immunohistochemistry in cats with ulcerative facial dermatitis, eosinophilic granuloma complex reaction patterns and mosquito bite hypersensitivity. *Vet Dermatol* **22**:521–527.

36

Bannoehr J, Brown JK, Shaw DJ et al. (2012) *Staphylococccus pseudintermedius* surface proteins SpsD and SpsO mediate adherence to ex vivo canine corneocytes. *Vet Dermatol* **23**:119–124.

References

Foster TJ (2009) Colonization and infection of the human host by staphylococci: adhesion, survival and immune evasion. *Vet Dermatol* 20:456–470.

Schmidt V, Nuttall T, Fazakerley J *et al.* (2009) *Staphylococcus intermedius* binding to immobilized fibrinogen, fibronectin and cytokeratin in vitro. *Vet Dermatol* 20:502–508.

Woolley KL, Kelly RF, Fazakerley J *et al.* (2008) Reduced in vitro adherence of *Staphylococcus* species to feline corneocytes compared to canine and human corneocytes. *Vet Dermatol* 19:1–6.

37
Fazakerley J, Nuttall T, Sales D *et al.* (2009) Staphylococcal colonization of mucosal and lesional skin sites in atopic and healthy dogs. *Vet Dermatol* 20:179–184.

Santoro D, Marsella R, Bunick D *et al.* (2011) Expression and distribution of canine antimicrobial peptides in the skin of healthy and atopic beagles. *Vet Immunol Immunopathol* 144:382–388.

Van Damme CM, Willemse T, van Dijk A *et al.* (2009) Altered cutaneous expression of beta-defensins in dogs with atopic dermatitis. *Mol Immunol* 46:2449–2455.

38
Gotzche PC, Johansen HK (2011) 'House dust mite control measures for asthma'. *Cochrane Library* 10:1–56.

Rosenkrantz W (2009) 'House dust mites and their control'. In: *Kirk's Current Veterinary Therapy XIV.* (eds JD Bonagura, DC Twedt) Saunders–Elsevier, St. Louis, pp. 425–427.

39
Chiaramonte D, Greco DS (2007) Feline adrenal disorders. *Clin Tech Small Anim Pract P* 22:26–31.

Helton-Rhodes K (1997) Cutaneous manifestations of hyperadrenocorticism. In: *Consultations in Feline Internal Medicine*, Vol. 3. (ed JR August) WB Saunders, Philadelphia, pp. 191–198.

Lien YH, Huang HP, Chang PH (2006) Iatrogenic hyperadrenocorticism in 12 cats. *J Am Anim Hosp Assoc* 42:414–423.

Lowe AD, Campbell KL, Graves T (2008) Glucocorticoids in the cat. *Vet Dermatol* 19:340–347.

40
Griffies JD, Mendelsohn CL, Rosenkrantz WE *et al.* (2004) Topical 0.1% tacrolimus for the treatment of discoid lupus erythematosus and atopic dermatitis. *Mol Immunol* 46:2449–2455.

pemphigus erythematosus in dogs. *J Am Anim Hosp Assoc* 40:29–41.

Oberkirchner U, Linder KE, Olivry T (2012) Successful treatment of a novel generalized variant of canine discoid lupus erythematosus with oral hydroxychloroquine. *Vet Dermatol* 23:23:65–70.

41
Frank LA, Hnilica KA, May ER (2005) Effects of sulfamethoxazole-trimethoprim on thyroid function in dogs. *Am J Vet Res* 66:256–259.

42
Ong PY, Boguniewicz M (2010) Investigational and unproven therapies in atopic dermatitis. *Immunol Allergy Clin N Am* 30:425–439.

43
Schinkel AH, Smit JJM, van Tellingen O *et al.* (1994) Disruption of the mouse mdr1a P-glycoprotein gene leads to a deficiency in the blood–brain barrier and to increased sensitivity to drugs. *Cell* 77:491–502.

44
Halliwell R (2006) Revised nomenclature for veterinary allergy. *Vet Immunol Immunopathol* 114:207–208.

Marsella R, Olivry T, Carlotti DN (2011) Current evidence of skin barrier dysfunction in human and canine atopic dermatitis. *Vet Dermatol* 22:239–248.

Olivry T, DeBoer DJ, Favrot C *et al.* (2010) Treatment of canine atopic dermatitis: 2010 clinical practice guidelines from the International Task Force on Canine Atopic Dermatitis. *Vet Dermatol* 21:233–248.

45
Scott DW (1987) Feline dermatology (1983–1985). 'The secret sits'. *J Am Anim Hosp Assoc* 23:255–274.

46
Page N, Paradis M, Lapointe J *et al.* (2003) Hereditary nasal hyperkeratosis in Labrador retrievers. *Vet Dermatol* 14:103–110.

47
Gross TL, Ihrke PJ, Walder EJ *et al.* (2005) *Skin Diseases of the Dog and Cat: Clinical and Histopathologic Diagnosis*, 2nd edn. Blackwell Publishing, Oxford.

Munday JS, Knight CG, Howe L (2010) The same papillomavirus is present in feline sarcoids from North America and New Zealand but not in any non-sarcoid feline samples. *J Vet Diagn Invest* 22:97–100.

Teifke JP, Kidney BA, Löhr CV *et al.* (2003) Detection of papillomavirus-DNA in mesenchymal tumour

cells and not in the hyperplastic epithelium of feline sarcoids *Vet Dermatol* 14:47–56.

48
Naidoo SL, Campbell DL, Miller LM *et al.* (2005) Necrotizing fasciitis: a review. *J Am Anim Hosp Assoc* 41:104–109.

Weese JS, Poma R, James F *et al.* (2009) *Staphylococcus pseud-intermedius* necrotizing fasciitis in a dog. *Can Vet J* 50:655–656.

Worth AJ, Marshall N, Thompson KG (2005) Necrotising fasciitis associated with *Escherichia coli* in a dog. *N Z Vet J* 53:257–260.

49
Greene CE(2006) *Infectious Diseases of the Cat and Dog*, 4th edn. Saunders–Elsevier, St. Lous.

50
Csiszer AB, Towle HA, Daly CM (2010) Successful treatment of necrotizing fasciitis in the hindlimb of a Great Dane. *J Am Anim Hosp Assoc* 46:433–438.

51
Simeonov R, Simeonova G (2008) Nucleomorphometric analysis of feline basal cell carcinomas. *Res Vet Sci* 84:440–443.

52
Preziosi DE, Gldschmidt MH, Greek JS *et al.*

(2003) Feline pemphigus foliaceus: a retrospective analysis of 57 cases. *Vet Dermatol* 14:313–321.

Rosenkrantz WS (2004) Pemphigus: current therapy. *Vet Dermatol* 15:90–98.

Tater KC, Olivry TO (2010) Canine and feline pemphigus foliaceus: improving your chances of a successful outcome. *Vet Med* 105:18–30.

53
Guardabasssi L, Schwarz S, Lloyd DH (2004) Pet animals as reservoirs of antimicrobial-resistant bacteria. *J Antimicrob Chemother* 54:321–332.

Van Duijkeren E, Kamphius M, van der Mije IC *et al.* (2011) Transmission of methicillin-resistant *Staphylococcus pseudintermedius* between infected dogs and cats and contact pets, humans and the environment in households and veterinary clinics. *Vet Microbiol* 150:338–343.

54
Onions AHS (1989) Prevention of mites in cultures. *World Federation for Culture Collections Technical Information Sheet 1.* http://www.cbs.knaw.nl/publications/mites.aspx.

55
Patterson AP, Campbell KL (2005) Managing anal furunculosis in dogs.

References

Comp Contin Educ Pract **27**:339–355.

Stanley BJ, Hauptman JG (2009) Long-term prospective evaluation of topically applied 0.1% tacrolimus ointment for treatment of perianal sinuses in dogs. *J Am Vet Med Assoc* **235**:397–404.

56

Coyner K (2010) Otomycosis due to *Aspergillus* spp. in a dog: case report and literature review. *Vet Dermatol* **21**:613–618.

Schultz RM, Johnson EG, Wisner ER *et al.* (2008) Clinicopathologic and diagnostic imaging characteristics of systemic aspergillosis in 30 dogs. *J Vet Intern Med* **22**:851–859.

58

Cohen JC, Hartman DG, Garofalo MJ *et al.* (2009) Comparison of closed chamber and open chamber evaporimetry. *Skin Res Technol* **15**:51–54.

Lau-Gillard PJ, Hill PB, Chesney CJ *et al.* (2010) Evaluation of a hand held evaporimeter (VapoMeter) for the measurement of transepidermal water loss in healthy dogs. *Vet Dermatol* **21**:136–145.

59

Bryan J, Frank L (2010) Food allergy in the cat: a diagnosis by elimination. *J Feline Med Surg* **12**:861–866.

Hobi S, Linek M, Marignac G *et al.* (2011) Clinical characteristics and causes of pruritus in cats: a multicentre study on feline hypersensitivity-associated dermatoses. *Vet Dermatol* **22**:406–413.

Jackson HA (2009) Food allergy in dogs – clinical signs and diagnosis. *EJCAP* **19**:230–233.

Raditic DM, Remillard RL, Tater KC (2011) ELISA testing for common food antigens in four dry dog foods used in dietary elimination trials. *J Anim Physiol Anim Nutr* **95**:90–97.

60

Griffies JD, Mendelsohn CL, Rosenkrantz WE *et al.* (2004) Topical 0.1% tacrolimus for the treatment of discoid lupus erythematosus and pemphigus erythematosus in dogs. *J Am Anim Hosp Assoc* **40**:29–41.

61

Raditic DM, Remillard RL, Tater KC (2011) ELISA testing for common food antigens in four dry dog foods used in dietary elimination trials. *J Anim Physiol Anim Nutr* **95**:90–97.

63

Isolauri E, Arvola T, Sütas Y *et al.* (2000) Probiotics in the management of atopic eczema. *Clin Exp Allergy* **30**:1604–1610.

Kalliomäki M, Salminen S, Arvilommi H *et al.* (2001) Probiotics in primary prevention of atopic disease: a randomized placebo-controlled trial. *Lancet* **357**:1076–1079.

Marsella R (2009) Evaluation of *Lactobacillus rhamnosus* strain GG for the prevention of atopic dermatitis in dogs. *Am J Vet Res* **70**:735–740.

Soccol CR, Vandenberghe L, Spier MR *et al.* (2010) The potential of probiotics: a review. *Food Technol Biotechnol* **48**:413–434.

64

Hicks MI, Elston DM (2009) Scabies. *Dermatol Ther* **22**:279–292.

66

Malik R, Wigney DI, Dawson D *et al.* (2000) Infection of the subcutis and skin of cats with rapidly growing mycobacteria: a review of microbiological and clinical findings. *J Feline Med Surg* **2**:35–48.

67

Olivry T, Bizikova P (2010) A systematic review of the evidence of reduced allergenicity and clinical benefit of food hydrolysates in dogs with cutaneous adverse food reactions. *Vet Dermatol* **21**:32–41.

References

68

Austel M, Hensel P, Jackson D et al. (2006) Evaluation of three different histamine concentrations in intradermal testing of normal cats and attempted determination of 'irritant' threshold concentrations for 48 allergens. Vet Dermatol 17:189–194.

Bauer CL, Hensel P, Austel M et al. (2010) Determination of irritant threshold concentrations to weeds, trees and grasses through serial dilutions in intradermal testing on healthy clinically nonallergic dogs. Vet Dermatol 21:192–197.

DeBoer DJ, Hillier A (2001) The ACVD task force on canine atopic dermatitis (XVI): laboratory evaluation of dogs with atopic dermatitis with serum-based 'allergy' tests. Vet Immunol Immunopathol 81:277–287.

Diesel A, DeBoer DJ (2011) Serum allergen-specific immunoglobulin E in atopic and healthy cats: comparison of a rapid screening immunoassay and complete-panel analysis. Vet Dermatol 22:39–45.

Hillier A, DeBoer DJ (2001) The ACVD task force on canine atopic dermatitis (XVII): intradermal testing. Vet Immunol Immunopathol 81:289–304.

Olivry T, Paps J (2011) Evaluation of the agreement between allergen-specific intradermal or IgE serological tests and a point-of-care immunodot assay in dogs with atopic dermatitis. Vet Dermatol 22:284–285.

69

Lange CE, Tobler K, Ackermann M et al. (2009) Three novel canine papillomaviruses support taxonomic clade formation. J Gen Virol 90:2615–2621.

Munday JS, O'Connor KI, Smits B (2011) Development of multiple pigmented viral plaques and squamous cell carcinomas in a dog infected by a novel papillomavirus. Vet Dermatol 22:104–110.

Tanabe C, Kano R, Nagata M et al. (2000) Molecular characteristics of cutaneous papillomavirus from the canine pigmented epidermal nevus. J Vet Med Sci 62:1189–1192.

Tobler K, Lange C, Carlotti DN et al. (2007) Detection of a novel papillomavirus in pigmented plaques of four pugs. Vet Dermatol 19:21–25.

70

DeBoer DJ, Hillier A (2001) The ACVD task force on canine atopic dermatitis (XVI): laboratory evaluation of dogs with atopic dermatitis with serum-based 'allergy' tests. Vet Immunol Immunopathol 81:277–287.

Wassom DL, Grieve RB (1998) In vitro measurement of canine and feline IgE: a review of FceR1a-based assays for detection of allergen-reactive IgE. Vet Dermatol 9:173–178.

71

Plant JD, Lund EM, Yang M (2011) A case-control study of the risk factors for canine juvenile-onset generalized demodicosis in the USA. Vet Dermatol 22:95–99.

72

Mueller RS (2004) Treatment protocols for demodicosis: an evidence-based review. Vet Dermatol 15:75–89.

76

Scott DW, Miller WH, Griffin CE (2001) Muller and Kirk's Small Animal Dermatology, 6th edn. WB Saunders, Philadelphia.

77

Salkin IF (1973) Dermatophyte Test Medium: evaluation with non-dermatophyte pathogens. App Microbiol 26:134–137.

Salkin IR, Pa AA, Kemna ME (1997) A new medium for the presumptive diagnosis

References

of dermatophytes. *J Clin Microbiol* 35:2660–2662.

Taplin D, Zais N, Rebell G *et al.* (1969) Isolation and recognition of dermatophytes on a new medium (DTM). *Arch Dermatol* 99:203–209.

78

Scott DW, Miller WH, Griffin CE (2001) *Muller and Kirk's Small Animal Dermatology*, 6th edn. WB Saunders, Philadelphia.

79

Graham PA, Refsal KR, Nachreiner RF (2007) Etiopathologic findings in canine hypothyroidism. *Vet Clin N Am* 37:617–631.

80

Ghubash R (2006) Parasitic miticidal therapy. *Clin Tech Small Anim Pract* 21:135–144.

83

Beningo KE, Scott D (2001) Idiopathic linear pustular acantholytic dermatosis in a young Brittany spaniel dog *Vet Dermatol* 12:209–213.

Scott DW (2003) Letter to the Editor: Canine idiopathic linear pustular acanthoyltic dermatosis: a second case. *Vet Dermatol* 14:275.

Weiss G, Shemer A, Trau H (2002) The Koebner phenomenon: review of the literature. *J Eur Acad Dermatol* 16:241–248.

87

Greer MB, Calhoun ML (1966) Anal sacs of the cat (*Felis domesticus*). *Am J Vet Res* 27:773–81.

Shoieb AM, Hanshaw DM (2009) Anal sac gland carcinoma in 64 cats in the United Kingdom (1995–2007). *Vet Pathol* 46:677–683.

88

Tey HL (2010) Approach to hypopigmentation disorders in adults. *Clin Exp Dermatol* 35:829–834.

89

Bowman DD, Hendrix CM, Lindsay DS *et al.* (2002) *Feline Clinical Parasitology*. Iowa State University Press, Ames, pp. 430–439.

Fiona MK, Poma J, Poma R (2010) Neurological manifestations of feline cuterebriasis. *Can Vet J* 51:213–215.

Glass EN, Cornetta AM, deLahunta A *et al.* (1998) Clinical and clinicopathologic features in 11 cats with *Cuterebra* larvae myiasis of the central nervous system. *J Vet Intern Med* 12:365–368.

Williams KJ, Summers BA, de LaHunta A (1998) Cerebrospinal cuterebriasis in cats and its association with feline ischemic encephalopathy. *Vet Pathol* 35:330–343.

91

Carlotti DN, Boulet M, Ducret J *et al.* (2009) The use of recombinant omega interferon therapy in canine atopic dermatitis: a double-blind controlled study. *Vet Dermatol* 20:405–411.

Gutzwiller MER (2010) Use of interferon omega for skin diseases. In: *Consultations in Feline Internal Medicine*, Vol. 6. (ed JR August) Saunders–Elsevier, St. Louis, pp. 382–389.

Yasukawa K, Saito S, Kubo T *et al.* (2010) Low-dose recombinant canine interferon-gamma for treatment of canine atopic dermatitis: an open randomized comparative trial of two doses. *Vet Dermatol* 21:42–49.

92

London CA, Dubilzeig RR, Vail DM *et al.* (1996) Evaluation of dogs and cats with tumors of the ear canal: 145 cases (1978–1992). *J Am Vet Med Assoc* 208:1413–1418.

93

Fitzgerald JR (2009) The *Staphylococcus intermedius* group of bacterial pathogens: species reclassification, pathogenesis, and emergence of methicillin resistance. *Vet Dermatol* 20:490–495.

94

Ahman SE, Bergström KE (2009) Cutaneous carriage of *Malassezia* species in healthy and seborrhoeic Sphynx cats and a comparison to carriage in Devon Rex cats. *J Feline Med Surg* 11:970–976.

Ahman S, Perrins N, Bond R (2007) Carriage of *Malassezia* spp. yeasts in healthy and seborrhoeic Devon Rex cats. *Med Mycol* 45:449–455.

Perrins N, Gaudiano F, Bond R (2007) Carriage of *Malassezia* spp. yeasts in cats with diabetes mellitus, hyperthyroidism and neoplasia. *Med Mycol* 45:541–546.

95

Credille KM, Lupton CJ, Kennis RA *et al.* (2002) What happens when a dog loses its puppy coat? Functional, developmental and breed related changes in the canine hair follicle. In: *Advances in Vet Dermatology*, Vol. 4. (eds KL Thoday, CS Foil, R Bond) Blackwell Publishing Ltd, Oxford, pp. 41–48.

96

Fourie LJ, Kok DJ, du Plessis A *et al.* (2007) Efficacy of a novel formulation of metaflumizone plus amitraz for the treatment of demodectic mange in dogs. *Vet Parasitol* 150:268–274.

Mueller RS, Meyer D, Bensignor E *et al.* (2010) Treatment of canine generalized demodicosis with a 'spot-on' formulation containing 10% moxidectin and 2.5% imidacloprid (Advocate®, Bayer Healthcare). In: *Advances in Veterinary Dermatology*, Vol. 6. (eds DJ DeBoer, VK Affolter, PB Hill) Wiley-Blackwell, West Sussex, pp. 181–186.

Rosenkrantz WS (2009) Efficacy of metaflumizone plus amitraz for treatment of juvenile and adult onset generalized demodicosis in dogs: pilot study of 24 dogs (Abstract). *Vet Dermatol* 20:227.

98

Wiemelt SP, Goldschmidt MH, Greek JS *et al.* (2004) A retrospective study comparing the histological features and response to treatment in two canine nasal dermatoses, DLE and MCP. *Vet Dermatol* 15:341–348.

99

Olivry T, DeBoer DJ, Favrot C *et al.* (2010) Treatment of canine atopic dermatitis: 2010 clinical practice guidelines from the International Task Force on Canine Atopic Dermatitis. *Vet Dermatol* 21:233–248.

101

Carlotti DN, personal communication.

Freeman K (2010) Update on the diagnosis and management of *Leishmania* spp. infections in dogs in the United States. *Top Companion Anim Med* 25:149–154.

Oliva G, Roura X, Crotti A *et al.* (2010) Guidelines for treatment of leishmaniasis in dogs. *J Am Vet Med Assoc* 236:1192–1198.

Trainor KE, Porter BF, Logan KS *et al.* (2010) Eight cases of feline cutaneous leishmaniasis in Texas. *Vet Pathol* 47:1076–1081.

102

Chang SW, Huang ZL (2006) Oral cimetidine adjuvant therapy for recalcitrant, diffuse conjunctival papillomatosis. *Cornea* 25:687–690.

Chern E, Cheng YW (2010) Treatment of recalcitrant periungual warts with cimetidine in pediatrics. *J Dermatolog Treat* 21:314–316.

Greene CE (2006) *Infectious Diseases of the Cat and Dog*, 4th edn. Saunders–Elsevier, St. Louis.

Kuntsi-Vaattovaara H, Verstraete FJM, Newsome JT *et al.* (2003) Resolution of persistent oral papillomatosis in a dog after treatment with a recombinant canine oral

References

papillomavirus vaccine. *Vet Comp Oncol* 1:57–63.

Yağci BB, Ural K, Ocal N et al. (2008) Azithromycin therapy of papillomatosis in dogs: a prospective, randomized, double-blinded, placebo-controlled clinical trial. *Vet Dermatol* 19:194–198.

103

Alexander JW (2009) History of the medical use of silver. *Surg Infect* 10:289–292.

Storm-Versloot MN, Vos CG, Ubbink DT et al. (2010) Topical silver for preventing wound infection (Review). *Cochrane Database Syst Rev* 17:1–112.

104

Asawanonda P, Taylor CR (1999) Wood's lamp in dermatology. *Int J Dermatol* 38:801–807.

Gupta LK, Singhi MK (2004) Wood's lamp. *Indian J Dermatol* 70:131–135.

Kefalidou S, Odia S, Gruseck E et al. (1997) Wood's lamp in *Microsporum canis*-positive patients. *Mycoses* 40:461–463.

Wolf FT (1957) Chemical nature of the fluorescent pigment produced in *Microsporum*-infected hair. *Nature* 180:860–861.

105

Holm KS, Morris DO, Gomez SM et al. (1999) Eosinophilic dermatitis with edema in nine dogs, compared with eosinophilic cellulitis in humans. *J Am Vet Med Assoc* 215:649–653.

Mauldin EA, Palmiero BS, Goldschmidt MH et al. (2006) Comparison of clinical history and dermatologic findings in 29 dogs with severe eosinophilic dermatitis: a retrospective analysis. *Vet Dermatol* 17:338–347.

106

Hobi S, Linek M, Marignac G et al. (2011) Clinical characteristics and causes of pruritus in cats: a multicentre study on feline hypersensitivity-associated dermatoses. *Vet Dermatol* 22:406–413.

107

Gross TL, Stannard AA, Yager JA (1997) An anatomical classification of folliculitis. *Vet Dermatol* 8:147–156.

Miller WH (1990) Color dilution alopecia in Doberman Pinschers with blue or fawn coat colors: a study on the incidence and histopathology of this disorder. *Vet Dermatol* 1:113–122.

108

Hardie EM, Linder KE, Pease AP (2008) Aural cholesteatoma in twenty dogs. *Vet Surg* 37:763–770.

Little CJ, Lane JG, Gibbs C et al. (1991) Inflammatory middle ear disease of the dog: the clinical and pathological features of cholesteatoma, a complication of otitis media. *Vet Rec* 128:319–322.

110

Galac S, Kars VJ, Voorhout G et al. (2008) ACTH-independent hyperadrenocorticism due to food-dependent hypercortisolemia in a dog: a case report. *Vet J* 177:141–143.

Galac S, Kooistra HS, Voorhout G et al. (2005) Hyperadrenocorticism in a dog due to ectopic secretion of adrenocorticotropic hormone. *Domest Anim Endocrinol* 28:338–348.

111

Kiupel M, Webster JD, Bailey KL et al. (2011) Proposal of a 2-tier histologic grading system for canine cutaneous mast cell tumors to more accurately predict biological behavior. *Vet Pathol* 48:147–155.

Welle MM, Bley CR, Howard J et al. (2008) Canine mast cell tumors: a review of the pathogenesis, clinical features, pathology and treatment. *Vet Dermatol* 19:321–339.

112

Brown CG, Graves TK (2007) Hyperadrenocorticism:

treating dogs. *Comp Contin Educ Pract* 29:132–134.

Kooistra HS, Galac S (2010) Recent advances in the diagnosis of Cushing's syndrome in dogs. *Vet Clin North Am Small Anim Pract* 40:259–267.

Zeugswetter F, Hoyer MT, Pagitz M *et al.* (2008) The desmopressin stimulation test in dogs with Cushing's syndrome. *Domest Anim Endocrinol* 34:254–260.

116

Lowe AD, Campbell KL, Graves T (2008) Glucocorticoids in the cat. *Vet Dermatol* 19:340–347.

Wildermuth BE, Griffin CE, Rosenkrantz WS (2012) Response of feline eosinophilic plaques and lip ulcers to amoxicillin trihydrate-clavulanate potassium therapy: a randomized, double-blind placebo-controlled prospective study. *Vet Dermatol* 23:110–118.

118

Bergman PJ, Camps-Palau MA, McKnight JA *et al.* (2006) Development of a xenogeneic DNA vaccine program for canine malignant melanoma at the Animal Medical Center. *Vaccine* 24:4582–4585.

Bergman PJ, McKnight J, Novosad A *et al.* (2003) Long-term survival of dogs with advanced malignant melanoma after DNA vaccination with xenogeneic human tyrosinase: a phase I trial. *Clin Cancer Res* 9:1284–1290.

Kim DY, Mauldin GE, Hosgood G *et al.* (2005) Perianal malignant melanoma in a dog. *J Vet Intern Med* 19:610–612.

119

Marconato L, Albanese F, Viacava P *et al.* (2007) Paraneoplastic alopecia associated with hepatocellular carcinoma in a cat. *Vet Dermatol* 18:267–271.

121

Casal ML, Straumann U, Sigg C *et al.* (1994) Congential hypotrichosis with thymic aplasia in nine Birman kittens. *J Am Anim Hosp Assoc* 30:600–602.

Vieira ALS, Ocarino NM, Boeloni JN *et al.* (2009) Congential oligodontia of the deciduous teeth and anodontia of the permanent teeth in a cat. *J Feline Med Surg* 11:156–158.

122

Burnett RC, Verneau W, Modiano JF *et al.* (2003) Diagnosis of canine lymphoid neoplasia using clonal rearrangements of antigen receptor genes. *Vet Pathol* 40:32–41.

De Mello Souza CH, Valli VEO *et al.* (2010) Immunohistochemical detection of retinoid receptors in tumors from 30 dogs diagnosed with cutaneous lymphoma. *J Vet Intern Med* 24:1112–1117.

Fontaine J, Bovens C, Bettenay S *et al.* (2009) Canine cutaneous epitheliotropic T-cell lymphoma: a review. *Vet Comp Oncol* 7:1–14.

123

Back DJ, Tjia JF (1991) Comparative effects of the antimycotic drugs ketoconazole, fluconazole, itraconazole and terbinafine on the metabolism of cyclosporin by human liver microsomes. *Brit J Clin Pharmacol* 32:624–626.

125

Loeffler A, Cobb MA, Bond R (2011) Comparison of a chlorhexidine and a benzoyl peroxide shampoo as sole treatment in canine superficial pyoderma. *Vet Rec* 169:249.

Löflath A, von Voigts-Rhetz A, Jaeger K *et al.* (2007) The efficacy of a commercial shampoo and whirlpooling in the treatment of canine pruritus: a double-blinded, randomized, placebo-controlled study. *Vet Dermatol* 18:427–431.

Ohmori K, Tanaka A, Makita Y *et al.* (2010) Pilot evaluation of the efficacy of shampoo

References

treatment with ultrapure soft water for canine pruritus. *Vet Dermatol* 21:477–483.

Young R, Buckley L, McEwan N *et al.* (2012) Comparative in vitro efficacy of antimicrobial shampoos: a pilot study. *Vet Dermatol* 23:36–40.

126
Affolter VK, Moore PF (2000) Canine cutaneous and systemic histiocytosis: reactive histiocytosis of dermal dendritic cells. *Am J Dermatopathol* 22:40–48.

Coomer AR, Liptak, JM (2008) Canine histiocytic diseases. *Comp Contin Educ Pract* 30:202–217.

Palmiero BS, Morris DO, Goldschmidt MH *et al.* (2007) Cutaneous reactive histiocytosis in dogs: a retrospective evaluation of 32 cases. *Vet Dermatol* 18:332–340.

128
Litster AL, Sorenmo KU (2006) Characterisation of the signalment, clinical and survival characteristics of 41 cats with mast cell neoplasia. *J Feline Med Surg* 8:177–183.

Rodriguez-Cariño C, Fondavila D, Segalés J *et al.* (2009) Expression of KIT receptor in feline cutaneous mast cell tumors. *Vet Pathol* 46:878–883.

Sabattini S, Bettini G (2010) Prognostic value of histologic and immunohistochemical features in feline cutaneous mast cell tumors. *Vet Pathol* 47:643–653.

130
Gil da Costa RM, Matos E, Rema A *et al.* (2007) CD117 immunoexpression in canine mast cell tumours: correlations with pathological variables and proliferation markers. *BMC Vet Res* 3:19.

Welle MM, Bley CR, Howard J *et al.* (2008) Canine mast cell tumors: a review of the pathogenesis, clinical features, pathology and treatment. *Vet Dermatol* 19:321–339.

132
Guardabassi L, Ghibaudo G, Damborg P (2010) In-vitro antimicrobial activity of a commercial ear antiseptic containing chlorhexidine and Tris-EDTA. *Vet Dermatol* 21:282–286.

Hawkins C, Harper D, Burch D *et al.* (2010) Topical treatment of *Pseudomonas aeruginosa* otitis of dogs with a bacteriophage mixture: a before/after clinical trial. *Vet Microbiol* 146:309–313.

Kaye D (1982) Enterococci. Biologic and epidemiologic characteristics and in vitro susceptibility. *Arch Intern Med* 142:2006–2009.

Stern-Bertholtz W, Sjöström L, Håkanson NW (2003) Primary secretory otitis media in the Cavalier King Charles spaniel: a review of 61 cases. *J Small Anim Pract* 44:253–256.

Swinney A, Fazakerley J, McEwan N *et al.* (2008) Comparative in vitro antimicrobial efficacy of commercial ear cleaners. *Vet Dermatol* 19:373–379.

Wildermuth BE, Griffin CE, Rosenkrantz WS *et al.* (2007) Susceptibility of *Pseudomonas* isolates from the ears and skin of dogs to enrofloxacin, marbofloxacin, and ciprofloxacin. *J Am Anim Hosp Assoc* 43:337–341.

133
Cerundolo R (2004) Generalized *Microsporum canis* dermatophytosis in six Yorkshire terrier dogs. *Vet Dermatol* 15:181–187.

Lewis DT, Foil CS, Hosgood G (1991) Epidemiology and clinical features of dermatophytosis in dogs and cats at Louisiana State University: 1981–90. *Vet Dermatol* 2:53–58.

134
Lee-Fowler TM, Cohn LA, DeClue AE *et al.* (2009) Evaluation of subcutaneous versus mucosal (intranasal) allergen-specific rush immunotherapy in experimental feline

asthma. *Vet Immunol Immunopathol* 129:49–56.

Mueller RS, Bettenay SV (2001) Evaluation of the safety of an abbreviated course of injections of allergen extracts (rush immunotherapy) for the treatment of dogs with atopic dermatitis. *Am J Vet Res* 62:307–310.

Mueller RS, Fieseler KV, Zabel S *et al.* (2004) Conventional and rush immunotherapy in canine atopic dermatitis. *Vet Dermatol* 15(s1):4 (abstract).

Reinero CR, Byerly JR, Berghaus RD *et al.* (2006) Rush immunotherapy in an experimental model of feline allergic asthma. *Vet Immunol Immunopathol* 110:141–153.

Reinero CR, Cohn LA, Delgado C *et al.* (2008) Adjuvanted rush immunotherapy using CpG oligodeoxynucleotides in experimental feline allergic asthma. *Vet Immunol Immunopathol* 121:241–250.

Trimmer AM, Griffen CE, Boord MJ *et al.* (2005) Rush allergen-specific immunotherapy protocol in feline atopic dermatitis: a pilot study of four cats. *Vet Dermatol* 16:324–329.

135

Olsson M, Meadows JRS, Truve K *et al.* (2011) A novel unstable duplication upstream of HAS2 predisposes to a breed-defining skin phenotype and a periodic fever syndrome in Chinese shar pei dogs. *PLoS Genetics* 7:3(1–11) Open Access.

136

Schwassman M, Logas D (2010) How to treat common parasites safely. In: *Consultations in Feline Internal Medicine*, Vol 6. (ed JR August) Saunders–Elsevier, St. Louis, pp. 390–398.

137

Angelakis E, Pulcini C, Waton J *et al.* (2010) Scalp eschar and neck lymphadenopathy caused by *Bartonella henselae* after tick bite. *Clin Infect Dis* 50:549–551.

Bechah Y, Socolovschi C, Raoult D (2011) Identification of rickettsial infections by using cutaneous swab specimens and PCR. *Emerg Infect Dis* 17:83–86.

Sliva N, Eremeeva ME, Rozental T *et al.* (2011) Eschar-associated spotted fever rickettsiosis, Bahi, Brazil. *Emerg Infect Dis* 17:275–278.

139

Michiels L, Day MJ, Snaps F *et al.* (2003) A retrospective study of non-specific rhinitis in 22 cats and the value of nasal cytology and histopathology. *J Feline Med Surg* 5:279–285.

142

Hinn AC, Olivry T, Luther PB (1998) Erythema multiforme, Stevens–Johnson syndrome, and toxic epidermal necrolysis in the dog: clinical classification, drug exposure, and histopathological correlations. *Vet Allergy Clin Immunol* 6:13–20.

Scott DW, Miller Jr WH (1999) Erythema multiforme in dogs and cats: literature review and case material from Cornell University College of Veterinary Medicine (1988–96). *Vet Dermatol* 10:297–309.

145

Baumgardner DJ, Paretsky DP, Yopp AC (1995) The epidemiology of blastomycosis in dogs: north central Wisconsin, USA. *J Med Vet Mycol* 33:171–176.

Foy DS, Trepanier LA (2010) Antifungal treatment of small animal veterinary patients. *Vet Clin North Am Small Anim Pract* 40:1171–1188.

Mazepa AS, Trepanier LA, Foy D (2011) Retrospective comparision of the efficacy of fluconazole or itraconazole for the treatment of systemic blastomycosis in dogs. *J Vet Intern Med* 25:440–445.

Spector D, Legendre AM, Wheat D *et al.* (2008)

References

Antigen and antibody testing for the diagnosis of blastomycosis in dogs. *J Vet Intern Med* 22:839–843.

146

Futagawa-Saito K, Makino S, Sunga F *et al*. (2009) Identification of the first exfoliative toxin in *Staphylococcus pseudointermedius*. *FEMS Microbiol Lett* 301:176–180.

Olivry T, Bizikova P (2009) A systematic review of the evidence of reduced allergenicity and clinical benefit of food hydrolysates in dogs with cutaneous adverse food reactions. *Vet Dermatol* 21:32–41.

147

Primavera G, Carrera M, Beradesca E *et al*. (2006) A double-blind, vehicle-controlled clinical study to evaluate the efficacy of MAS065D (XClair), a hyaluronic acid-based formulation, in the management of radiation-induced dermatitis. *Cutan Ocul Toxicol* 25:165–171.

149

Park C, Yoo JH, Kim HJ *et al*. (2010) Combination of cyclosporin A and prednisolone for juvenile cellulitis concurrent with hindlimb paresis in 3 English cocker spaniel puppies. *Can Vet J* 51:1265–1268.

150

Corfield GS, Burrows AK, Imani P *et al*. (2008) The method of application and short-term results of tympanostomy tubes for the treatment of primary secretory otitis media in three Cavalier King Charles Spaniel dogs. *Aust Vet J* 86:88–94.

Stern-Bertholtz W, Sjöström L, Håkanson NW (2003) Primary secretory otitis media in the Cavalier King Charles spaniel: a review of 61 cases. *J Small Anim Pract* 44:253–256.

151

Oberkirchner U, Linder KE, Dunston S *et al*. (2011) Metaflumizone-amitraz (Promeris)-associated pustular acantholytic dermatitis in 22 dogs: evidence suggests contact drug-triggered pemphigus foliaceus. *Vet Dermatol* 22:436–448.

153

Woolley KL, Kelly RF, Fazakerley J *et al*. (2008) Reduced in vitro adherence of *Staphylococcus* species to feline corneocytes compared to canine and human corneocytes. *Vet Dermatol* 19:1–6.

154

Kovalik M, Thoday KL, Berry J *et al*. (2012) Prednisolone therapy for atopic dermatitis is less effective in dogs with lower pretreatment serum 25-hydroxyvitamin D concentrations. *Vet Dermatol* 23:125–130.

Searing DA, Leung DYM (2010) Vitamin D in atopic dermatitis, asthma and allergic diseases. *Immunol Allergy Clin North Am* 30:397–409.

157

Bhatti SF, Duchateau L, Okkens AC *et al*. (2006) Treatment of growth hormone excess in dogs with the progesterone receptor antagonist aglépristone. *Theriogenology* 66:797–803.

158

Gross TL, Ihrke PJ, Walder EJ *et al*. (2005) *Skin Diseases of the Dog and Cat: Clinical and Histopathologic Diagnosis*, 2nd edn. Blackwell Publishing, Oxford.

159

Blot C, Kodjo A, Reynaude MC *et al*. (2003) Efficacy of selamectin administered topically in the treatment of feline otoacariosis. *Vet Parasitol* 112:241–247.

Otranto D, Milillo P, Mesto P *et al*. (2004) *Otodectes cynotis* (Acari: Psoroptidae): examination of survival off-the-host under natural and laboratory conditions. *Exp AppAcarol* 32:171–180.

Scott DW, Miller WH, Griffin CE (2001) *Muller*

and Kirk's Small Animal Dermatology, 6th edn. WB Saunders, Philadelphia.

161
Mueller RS, Rosychuk RA, Jonas LD (2003) A retrospective study regarding the treatment of lupoid onychodystrophy in 30 dogs and literature review. *J Am Anim Hosp Assoc* **39:**139–150.

162
Moriello KA, DeBoer DJ, Volk LM *et al.* (2004) Development of an in vitro, isolated infected spore testing model for disinfectant testing of *Microsporum canis* isolates. *Vet Dermatol* **15:**175–180.
White-Weithers N, Medleau L (1995) Evaluation of topical therapies for the treatment of dermatophyte infected hairs from dogs and cat. *J Am Anim Hosp Assoc* **31:**250–253.

163
Kirby KA, Wheeler JL, Farese JP *et al.* (2009) Surgical views: vacuum-assisted wound closure: application and mechanism of action. *Comp Contin Educ Pract* **31:**568–576.
Kirby KA, Wheeler JL, Farese JP *et al.* (2010) Surgical views: vacuum-assisted wound closure: clinical applications. *Comp Contin Educ Pract* **32:**E1–E7.

165
Edwards ML (2010) Hyperbaric oxygen therapy. Part 2: application in disease. *J Vet Emerg Crit Care* **20:**289–297.

166
Felsten LM, Alikhan A, Petronic-Rosic V (2011) Vitiligo. A comprehensive overview: Part II: Treatment options and approach to treatment. *J Am Acad Dermatol* **65:**493–514.

167
Kelley LS, Flynn-Lurie AK, House RA *et al.* (2010) Safety and tolerability of 0.1% tacrolimus solution applied to the external ear canals of atopic beagle dogs without otitis. *Vet Dermatol* **21:**554–565.
Kesser BW (2011) Assessment and management of chronic otitis externa. *Curr Opin Otolaryngol Head Neck Surg* **19:**341–347.

169
Gnirs K, Prélaud P (2005) Cutaneous manifestations of neurological diseases: review of neuro-pathophysiology and diseases causing pruritus. *Vet Dermatol* **16:**137–146.
Marino DJ (2011) Chiari-like malformation: the scratching dog only a neurosurgeon can help. In: *Proc 2011 North American Veterinary*

Dermatology Forum, pp. 117–125.
Metz M, Grundmann S, Ständer S (2011) Pruritus: an overview of current concepts. *Vet Dermatol* **22:**121–131.

172
Bizikova P, Dean GA, Hashimoto T *et al.* (2011) Desmocollin-1 is a major autoantigen in canine pemphigus foliaceus. *Vet Dermatol* **22:**299 (abstract).
Olivry T, Linder KE (2009) Dermatoses affecting desmosomes in animals: a mechanistic review of acantholytic blistering skin diseases. *Vet Dermatol* **20:**313–326.

174
Hillier A, Cole LK, Kwochka KW *et al.* (2002) Late-phase reactions to intradermal testing with *Dermatophagoides farinae* in healthy dogs and dogs with house dust mite-induced atopic dermatitis. *Am J Vet Res* **63:**69–73.

175
Ahman S, Perrins N, Bond R (2007) Carriage of *Malassezia* spp. yeasts in healthy and seborrhoeic Devon Rex cats. *Med Mycol* **45:**449–455.
Ahman SE, Bergström KE (2009) Cutaneous carriage of *Malassezia* species in healthy and seborrhoeic Sphynx cats

References

and a comparison to carriage in Devon Rex cats. *J Feline Med Surg* 11:970–976.

Bensignor E (2010) Treatment of *Malassezia* overgrowth with itraconazole in 15 cats. *Vet Rec* 167:1011–1012.

Bond R, Stevens K, Perrins N *et al.* (2008) Carriage of *Malassezia* spp. yeasts in Cornish Rex, Devon Rex and domestic short-haired cats: a cross-sectional survey. *Vet Dermatol* 19:299–304.

Colombo S, Nardoni S, Cornegliani L *et al.* (2007) Prevalence of *Malassezia* spp. yeasts in feline nail folds: a cytological and mycological study. *Vet Dermatol* 18:278–283.

Perrins N, Gaudiano F, Bond R (2007) Carriage of *Malassezia* spp. yeasts in cats with diabetes mellitus, hyperthyroidism and neoplasia. *Med Mycol* 45:541–546.

Shokri H, Khosravi A, Rad M *et al.* (2010) Occurrence of *Malassezia* species in Persian and domestic short-hair cats with and without otitis externa. *J Vet Med Sci* 72:293–296.

178

De Mello Souza CH, Valli VEO *et al.* (2010) Immunohistochemical detection of retinoid receptors in tumors from 30 dogs diagnosed with cutaneous lymphoma. *J*

Vet Intern Med 24:1112–1117.

Fontaine J, Bovens C, Bettenay S *et al.* (2009) Canine cutaneous epitheliotropic T-cell lymphoma: a review. *Vet Comp Oncol* 7:1–14.

Rechner KN, Weeks KJ, Pruitt AF (2011) Total skin electron therapy technique for the canine patient. *Vet Radiol Ultrasound* 52:345–352.

179

Mueller RS, Bensignor E, Ferrer L *et al.* (2012) Treatment of dermodicosis in dogs: 2011 clinical practice guidelines. *Vet Dermatol* 23:86–96.

182

Cerundolo R, Lloyd DH, Persechino A *et al.* (2004) Treatment of canine alopecia X with trilostane. *Vet Dermatol* 15:285–293.

Frank LA (2007) Oestrogen receptor antagonist and hair regrowth in dogs with hair cycle arrest (alopecia X). *Vet Dermatol* 18:63–66.

Frank LA, Donnell RL, Kania SA (2006) Oestrogen receptor evaluation in Pomeranian dogs with hair cycle arrest (alopecia X) on melatonin supplementation. *Vet Dermatol* 17:252–258.

Frank LA, Hnilica KA, Oliver JW (2004) Adrenal steroid hormone concentrations in dogs

with hair cycle arrest (alopecia X) before and during treatment with melatonin and mitotane. *Vet Dermatol* 15:278–284.

Leone F, Cerundolo R, Vercelli A *et al.* (2005) The use of trilostane for the treatment of alopecia X in Alaskan malamutes. *J Am Anim Hosp Assoc* 41:336–342.

Mausberg EM, Drögemüller C, Dolf G *et al.* (2008) Exclusion of patched homolog 2 (PTCH2) as a candidate gene for alopecia X in Pomeranians and Keeshonden. *Vet Rec* 163:121–123.

184

Favrot C, Steffan J, Seewald W *et al.* (2010) A prospective study on the clinical features of chronic atopic dermatitis and its diagnosis. *Vet Dermatol* 21:23–31.

185

Gilor C, Ridgway MD, Singh K (2011) DIC and granulomatous vasculitis in a dog with disseminated histoplasmosis. *J Am Anim Hosp Assoc* 47:e26–30.

Morris DO, Beale KM (1999) Cutaneous vasculitis and vasculopathy. *Vet Clin North Am Small Anim Pract* 29:1325–1335.

186
Candi E, Schmidt R, Melino G (2005) The cornified envelope: a model of cell death in the skin. *Nat Rev Mol Cell Biol* **6**:328–340.

187
Halliwell R (2006) Revised nomenclature for veterinary allergy. *Vet Immunol Immunopathol* **114**:207–208.

Hobi S, Linek M, Marignac G *et al.* (2011) Clinical characteristics and causes of pruritus in cats: a multicentre study on feline hypersensitivity-associated dermatoses. *Vet Dermatol* **22**:406–413.

Reedy LM (1982) Results of allergy testing and hyposensitization in selected feline skin diseases. *J Am Anim Hosp Assoc* **18**:618–623.

Reinero CR (2009) Feline immunoglobulin E: historical perspective, diagnostics and clinical relevance. *Vet Immunol Immunopathol* **132**:13–20.

190
Gill VL, Bergman PJ, Baer KE *et al.* (2008) Use of imiquimod 5% cream (Aldara) in cats with mulitcentric squamous cell carcinoma in situ: 12 cases (2002–2005). *Vet Comp Oncol* **6**:55–64.

Peters-Kennedy J, Scott DW, Miller WH (2008) Apparent clinical resolution of pinnal actinic keratoses and squamous cell carcinoma in a cat using topical imiquimod 5% cream. *J Feline Med Surg* **10**:593–599.

Torres SM, Malone ED, White SD *et al.* (2010) The efficacy of imiquimod 5% cream (Aldara®) in the treatment of aural plaque in horses: a pilot open-label clinical trial. *Vet Dermatol* **21**:503–509.

Whilhelm S, Degorce–Rubiales, Godson D *et al.* (2006) Clinical, histological and immunohistochemical study of feline viral plaques and bowenoid in situ carcinomas. *Vet Dermatol* **17**:424–431.

191
Woolley KL, Kelly RF, Fazakerley J *et al.* (2008) Reduced in vitro adherence of *Staphylococcus* species to feline corneocytes compared to canine and human corneocytes. *Vet Dermatol* **19**:1–6.

192
Malik R, Lessels NS, Webb S *et al.* (2009) Treatment of feline herpesvirus-1-associated disease in cats with famciclovir and related drugs. *J Feline Med Surg* **11**:40–48.

195
Desch CE, Hillier A (2003) *Demodex injai*: a new species of hair follicle mite (Acari: Demodecidae) from the domestic dog (Canidae). *J Med Entomol* **40**:146–149.

Ordeix L, Bardagi M, Scarampella F *et al.* (2009) *Demodex injai* infestation and dorsal greasy skin and hair in eight wirehaired fox terrier dogs. *Vet Dermatol* **20**:267–272.

196
Gupta D, Agarwal R, Aggarwal AN *et al.* (2011) Immune responses to mycobacterial antigens in sarcoidosis: a systematic review. *Indian J Chest Dis Allied Sci* **53**:41–49.

197
Burrows A, Mason KV (1994) Observations on the pathogenesis and treatment of lichenoid-psoriasiform dermatitis of Springer Spaniels. In: *Proc 10ᵗʰ AAVD/ACVD Meeting, Charleston*, p. 81.

Guttman-Yassky E, Nograles KE, Krueger JG (2011) Contrasting pathogenesis of atopic dermatitis and psoriasis. Part I: clinical and pathologic concepts. *J Allergy Clin Immunol* **127**:1110–1118.

Mason KV, Halliwell REW, McDougal BJ (1986) Characterization of lichenoid-psoriasiform dermatosis of Springer Spaniels. *J Am Vet Med Assoc* **189**:897–901.

References

Werner AH (2003) Psoriasiform-lichenoid-like dermatosis in three dogs treated with microemulsified cyclosporine A. *J Am Vet Med Assoc* **223**:1013–1016.

199

Jackson HA (2004) Eleven cases of cutaneous lupus erythematosus in Shetland sheepdogs and rough collies: clinical management and prognosis. *Vet Dermatol* **15**:37–41.

Jackson HA, Olivry T (2001) Ulcerative dermatosis of the Shetland sheepdog and rough collie dog may represent a novel vesicular variant of cutaneous lupus erythematosus. *Vet Dermatol* **12**:19–27.

Jackson HA, Olivry T, Berget F *et al.* (2004) Immunopathology of vesicular cutaneous erythematosus in the rough collie and Shetland sheepdog: a canine homologue of subacute cutaneous lupus erythematosus in humans. *Vet Dermatol* **15**:230–239.

200

Guilliard MJ, Segboer I, Shearer DH (2010) Corns in dogs; signalment, possible aetiology and response to surgical treatment. *J Small Anim Pract* **51**:162–168.

201

Bettenay SV, Lappin MR, Mueller RS (2007) An immunohistochemical and polymerase chain reaction evaluation of feline plasmacytic pododermatitis. *Vet Pathol* **44**:80–83.

Declercq J, DeBosschere H (2010) Nasal swelling due to plasma cell infiltrate in a cat without plasma cell pododermatitis. *Vet Dermatol* **21**:412–414.

Patel A, Forsythe P (2008) Feline plasma cell pododermatitis. In: *Saunder's Solutions in Veterinary Practice: Small Animal Dermatology*. Saunders–Elsevier, Edinburgh, p. 310.

Simon M, Horvath C, Pauley D *et al.* (1993) Plasma cell pododermatits in immunodeficiency virus-infected cats. *Vet Pathol* **30**:477.

202

Bissonnette S, Paradis M, Daneau I *et al.* (2008) The *ABCB1-1*D mutation is not responsible for subchronic neurotoxicity seen in dogs of non-collie breeds following macrocyclic lactone treatment for generalized demodicosis. *Vet Dermatol* **20**:60–66.

Hugnet C, Bentjen SA, Mealey KL (2004) Frequency of the mutant MDR1 allele associated with multidrug sensitivity in a sample of collies from France. *J Vet Pharmacol Therap* **27**:227–229.

Mealey KL (2004) Therapeutic implications of the MDR-1 gene. *J Vet Pharmacol Therap* **27**:257–264.

Novotny MJ, Krautmann MJ, Ehrhart JC *et al.* (2000) Safety of selamectin in dogs. *Vet Parasitol* **91**:377–391.

Paul AJ, Tranquilli WJ, Hutchens DE (2000) Safety of moxidectin in avermectin-sensitive Collies. *Am J Vet Res* **6**:482–483.

204

Hobi S, Linek M, Marignac G *et al.* (2011) Clinical characteristics and causes of pruritus in cats: a multicentre study on feline hypersensitivity-associated dermatoses. *Vet Dermatol* **22**:406–413.

205

Kim H-J, Kang M-H, Kim J-H *et al.* (2011) Sterile panniculitis in dogs: new diagnostic findings and alternative treatments. *Vet Dermatol* **22**:352–359.

206

Rush JE, Freeman LM, Fenollosa NK *et al.* (2002) Population and survival characteristics of cats with hypertrophic cardiomyopathy: 260 cases (1990–1999). *J Am Vet Med Assoc* **220**:202–207.

Smith SA, Tobias AH, Fine DM *et al.* (2004) Corticosteroid-associated congestive heart failure in 12 cats. *Int J App Res Vet Med* **2**:159–170.

208

Duckworth DH, Gulig PA (2002) Bacteriophages: potential treatment for bacterial infections. *Biodrugs* **16**:57–62.

Gu J, Xu W, Lei L *et al.* (2011) LysGH15, a novel bacteriophage lysin, protects a murine bacteremia model efficiently against lethal methicillin-resistant *Staphylococcus aureus* infection. *J Clin Microbiol* **49**:111–117.

Hawkins C, Harper D, Burch D *et al.* (2010) Topical treatment of *Pseudomonas aeruginosa* otitis of dogs with a bacteriophage mixture: a before/after clinical trial. *Vet Microbiol* **146**:309–313.

Kumari S, Harjai K, Chhibber S (2009) Efficacy of bacteriophage treatment in murine burn wound infection induced by *Klebsiella pneumoniae*. *J Microbiol Biotech* **19**:622–628.

Kumari S, Harjai K, Chhibber S (2011) Bacteriophage versus antimicrobial agents for the treatment of murine burn wound infection caused by *Klebsiella pneumoniae* B5055. *J Med Microbiol* **60**:205–210.

Malik R, Chhibber S (2009) Protection with bacteriophage KØ1 against fatal *Klebsiella pneumoniae*-induced burn wound infection in mice. *J Microbiol Immunol Infect* **42**:134–140.

Pastagia M, Euler C, Chahales P *et al.* (2011) A novel chimeric lysin shows superiority to mupirocin for skin decolonization of methicillin-resistant and -sensitive *Staphylococcus aureus* strains. *Antimicrob Agents Chemother* **55**:738–744.

Sivera-Marza JA, Soothill JS, Boydell P *et al.* (2006) Multiplication of therapeutically administered bacteriophages in *Pseudomonas aeruginosa* infected patients. *Burns* **32**:644–646.

209

Bellini MH, Caldini ET, Scapinelli MP *et al.* (2009) Increased elastic microfibrils and thickening of fibroblastic nuclear lamina in canine cutaneous asthenia. *Vet Dermatol* **20**:139–143.

Prontera P, Belcastro V, Calabresi P *et al.* (2010) Myostatin depletion: a therapy for Ehlers–Danlos syndrome? *Ann Neurol* **67**:147–148.

Rombaut L, Malfait F, Cools A *et al.* (2010) Musculoskeletal complaints, physical activity, and health-related quality of life among patients with Ehlers–Danlos syndrome hypermobility type. *Disabil Rehabil* **32**:1339–1345.

210

Declercq J, DeBosschere H (2010) Nasal swelling due to plasma cell infiltrate in a cat without plasma cell pododermatitis. *Vet Dermatol* **21**:412–414.

215

Oberkirchner U, Linder KE, Dunston S *et al.* (2011) Metaflumizone-amitraz (Promeris)-associated pustular acantholytic dermatitis in 22 dogs: evidence suggests contact drug-triggered pemphigus foliaceus. *Vet Dermatol* **22**:436–448.

Rybníček J, Hill PB (2007) Suspected polymyxin B-induced pemphigus vulgaris in a dog. *Vet Dermatol* **18**:165–170.

White SD, Carlotti DN, Pin D *et al.* (2002) Putative drug-related pemphigus foliaceus in four dogs. *Vet Dermatol* **13**:195–202.

Wolf R, Tamir A, Brenner S (1991) Drug-induced versus drug-triggered pemphigus. *Dermatologica* **182**:207–210.

216

Anthony RM, Kobayashi T, Wermeling F *et al.* (2011) Intravenous gammaglobulin suppresses inflammation through a novel T(H)2 pathway. *Nature* **475**:110–113.

References

Bianco D, Armstrong PJ, Washabau RJ (2009) A prospective, randomized, double-blinded, placebo-controlled study of human intravenous immunoglobulin for the acute management of presumptive primary immune-mediated thrombocytopenia in dogs. *J Vet Intern Med* 23:1071–1078.

Kellerman DL, Bruyette DS (1997) Intravenous human immunoglobulin for the treatment of immune-mediated hemolytic anemia in 13 dogs. *J Vet Intern Med* 11:327–332.

Rahilly LJ, Keating JH, O'Toole TE (2006) The use of intravenous human immunoglobulin in treatment of severe pemphigus foliaceus in a dog. *J Vet Intern Med* 20:1483–1486.

Rosenkrantz WS (2004) Pemphigus: current therapy. *Vet Dermatol* 15:90–98.

Smith SD, Dennington PM, Cooper A (2010) The use of intravenous immunoglobulin for treatment of dermatological conditions in Australia: a review. *Aust J Dermatol* 51:227–237.

Trotman TK, Phillips H, Fordyce H *et al.* (2006) Treatment of severe adverse cutaneous drug reactions with human intravenous immunoglobulin in two dogs. *J Am Anim Hosp Assoc* 42:312–320.

217

Cobb MA, Edwards HJ, Jagger TD *et al.* (2005) Topical fusidic acid/betamethasone-containing gel compared to systemic therapy in the treatment of canine acute moist dermatitis. *Vet J* 169:276–280.

Holm BR, Rest JR, Seewald W (2004) A prospective study of the clinical findings, treatment and histopathology of 44 cases of pyotraumatic dermatitis. *Vet Dermatol* 15:369–376.

218

Mueller RS, Bergvall K, Besignor E *et al.* (2012) A review of topical therapy for skin infections with bacteria and yeast. *Vet Dermatol* 23:380–341.

Negre A, Bensignor E, Guillot J (2009) Evidence-based veterinary dermatology: a systematic review of interventions for *Malassezia* dermatitis in dogs. *Vet Dermatol* 20:1–12.

219

Patel A (2006) Bacterial pyoderma. In: *Consultations in Feline Internal Medicine*, Vol. 5. (ed JR August) Elsevier, St. Louis, pp. 251–259.

Wildermuth BE, Griffin CE, Rosenkrantz WS (2006) Feline pyoderma therapy. *Clin Tech Small Anim Pract* 21:150–156.

221

Cadiergues MC, Patel A, Shearer DH *et al.* (2008) Cornification defect in the golden retriever: clinical, histopathological, ultrastructural and genetic characterisation. *Vet Dermatol* 19:120–129.

Credille KM, Barnhart KF, Minor JS *et al.* (2005) Mild recessive epidermolytic hyperkeratosis associated with a novel keratin 10 donor splice-site mutation in a family of Norfolk terrier dogs. *Brit J Dermatol* 153:51–58.

Credille KM, Minor JS, Barnhart KF *et al.* (2009) Transglutaminase 1-deficient recessive lamellar ichthyosis associated with a LINE-1 insertion in Jack Russell terrier dogs. *Brit J Dermatol* 161:265–272.

Grall A, Guaguere E, Planchais S *et al.* (2012) PNPLA1 mutations cause autosomal recessive congenital ichthyosis in golden retriever dogs and humans. *Nat Genet* 44:140–147.

Guaguere E, Bensignor E, Küry S *et al.* (2009) Clinical, histopathological and genetic data of ichthyosis in the golden retriever: a prospective study. *J Small Anim Pract* 50:227–235.

223

Campbell GA, Crow D (2010) Severe zinc responsive skin dermatosis in a litter of Pharaoh Hounds. *J Vet Diagn Invest* 22:663–666.

224

Yang S, Liu C, Hsu C et al. (2007) Use of chemical ablation with trichloroacetic acid to treat apocrine hidrocystomas in a cat. *J Am Vet Med Assoc* 230:1170–1173.

225

Diesel A, Moriello KA (2008) A busy clinician's review of cyclosporine. *Vet Med* 103:266–273.

Galgut BI, Janardhan KS, Grondin TM et al. (2010) Detection of *Neospora caninum* tachyzoites in cerebrospinal fluid of a dog following prednisone and cyclosporine therapy. *Vet Clin Pathol* 39:386–390.

Guaguère E, Steffan J, Olivry T (2004) Cyclosporin A: a new drug in the field of canine dermatology. *Vet Dermatol* 15:61–74.

Kim H-J, Kang M-H, Kim J-H et al. (2011) Sterile panniculitis in dogs: new diagnostic findings and alternative treatments. *Vet Dermatol* 22:352–359.

Kovalik M, Thoday KL, Handel IG et al. (2011) Ciclosporin A therapy is associated with disturbances in glucose metabolism in dogs with atopic dermatitis. *Vet Dermatol* 22:173–180.

MacNeill AL, Steeil JC, Dossin O et al. (2010) Disseminated nocardiosis caused by *Nocardia abscessus* in a dog. *Vet Clin Pathol* 39:381–385.

Palmiero BS, Morris DO, Goldschmidt MH et al. (2007) Cutaneous reactive histiocytosis in dogs: a retrospective evaluation of 32 cases. *Vet Dermatol* 18:332–340.

Park C, Yoo JH, Kim HJ et al. (2010) Combination of cyclosporin A and prednisolone for juvenile cellulitis concurrent with hindlimb paresis in 3 English cocker spaniel puppies. *Can Vet J* 51:1265–1268.

Robson D (2003) Review of the pharmacokinetics, interactions and adverse reactions of cyclosporine in people, dogs, and cats. *Vet Rec* 152:739–748.

Robson D, Burton GG (2003) Cyclosporin: applications in small animal dermatology. *Vet Dermatol* 14:1–9.

228

Toma S, Cornegliani L, Persico P et al. (2006) Comparison of 4 fixation and staining methods for the cytologic evaluation of ear canals with clinical evidence of ceruminous otitis externa. *Vet Clin Pathol* 35:194–198.

229

Bardagi M, Lloret A, Fondati A et al. (2007) Neutrophilic dermatosis resembling pyoderma gangrenosum in a dog with polyarthritis. *J Small Anim Pract* 48:229–232.

Gains MJ, Morency A, Sauvé F et al. (2010) Canine sterile neutrophilic dermatitis (resembling Sweet's syndrome) in a Dachshund. *Can Vet J* 51:1397–1399.

Johnson CS, May ER, Myers RK et al. (2009) Extracutaneous neutrophilic inflammation in a dog with lesions resembling Sweet's syndrome. *Vet Dermatol* 20:200–205.

230

Clark LA, Credille KM, Murphy KE et al. (2005) Linkage of dermatomyositis in the Shetland Sheepdog to chromosome 35. *Vet Dermatol* 16:392–394.

Haupt KH, Prieur DJ, Moore MP et al. (1985) Familial canine dermatomyositis: clinical, electrodiagnostic, and genetic studies. *Am J Vet Res* 46:1861–1869.

Rees CA, Boothe DM (2003) Therapeutic response to pentoxifylline and its active metabolites in dogs with familial canine dermatomyositis. *Vet Therap* 4:234–241.

Wahl JM, Clark LA, Skalli O et al. (2008) Analysis of gene transcript profiling

References

and immunobiology in Shetland sheepdogs with dermatomyositis. *Vet Dermatol* **19**:52–58.

234
Mauldin EA, Tess TA, Goldschmidt MH (2007) Proliferative and necrotizing otitis externa in four cats. *Vet Dermatol* **18**:370–377.

Vidémont E, Pin D (2010) Proliferative and necrotising otitis in a kitten: first demonstration of T-cell-mediated apoptosis. *J Small Anim Pract* **51**:599–603.

235
Frazer MM, Schick AE, Lewis TP *et al.* (2010) Sebaceous adenitis in Havanese dogs: a retrospective study on the clinical presentation and incidence. *Vet Dermatol* **22**:267–274.

236
AVMA Web Site. *Vaccine-associated Feline Sarcoma Task Force Guidelines: Diagnosis and Management of Suspected Sarcoma.* (http://www.avma.org/vafst)

237
Gross TL, Ihrke PJ, Walder EJ *et al.* (2005) *Skin Diseases of the Dog and Cat: Clinical and Histopathologic Diagnosis*, 2nd edn. Blackwell Publishing, Oxford.

238
Eom K, Kwak H, Kang H *et al.* (2008) Virtual CT otoscopy of the middle ear and ossicles in dogs. *Vet Radiol Ultrasound* **49**:545–550.

Rohleder JJ, Jones JC, Duncan RB *et al.* (2006) Comparative performance of radiography and computed tomography in the diagnosis of middle ear disease in 31 dogs. *Vet Radiol Ultrasound* **47**:45–52.

239
Veraldi S, Girgenti V, Dassoni F *et al.* (2009) Erysipeloid: a review. *Clin Exp Dermatol* **34**:859–862.

Wang Q, Chang BJ, Riley TV (2010) *Erysipelothrix rhusiopathiae*. *Vet Microbiol* **140**:405–417.

240
Binford GJ, Bodner MR, Cordes MHJ *et al.* (2009) Molecular evolution, functional variation, and proposed nomenclature of the gene family that includes sphingomyelinase D in sicariid spider venoms. *Mol Biol Evol* **26**:547–566.

243
Fondati A, De Lucia M, Furiani N *et al.* (2010) Prevalence of *Demodex canis*-positive healthy dogs at trichoscopic examination. *Vet Dermatol* **21**:146–151.

Saridomichelakis MN, Koutinas AF, Farmaki R *et al.* (2007) Relative sensitivity of hair pluckings and exudate microscopy for the diagnosis of canine demodicosis. *Vet Dermatol* **18**:138–141.

245
Hillier A, Alcorn JR, Cole L *et al.* (2006) Pyoderma caused by *Pseudomonas aeruginosa* in dogs: 20 cases. *Vet Dermatol* **17**:432–439.

Index

Index

Index

Index

Index

Index

Index

Printed and bound by CPI Group (UK) Ltd, Croydon, CR0 4YY

23/10/2024

01777705-0001